Simplified
Vectorcardiography

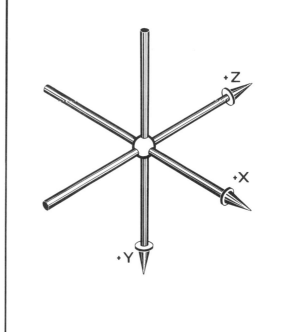

Simplified Vectorcardiography

JOZEF WARTAK, M.D., B.Sc.

Research Cardiologist,
Department of Medicine, Queen's University,
Kingston, Ontario

337 Illustrations

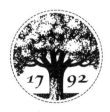

J. B. Lippincott Company

Philadelphia • Toronto

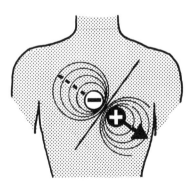

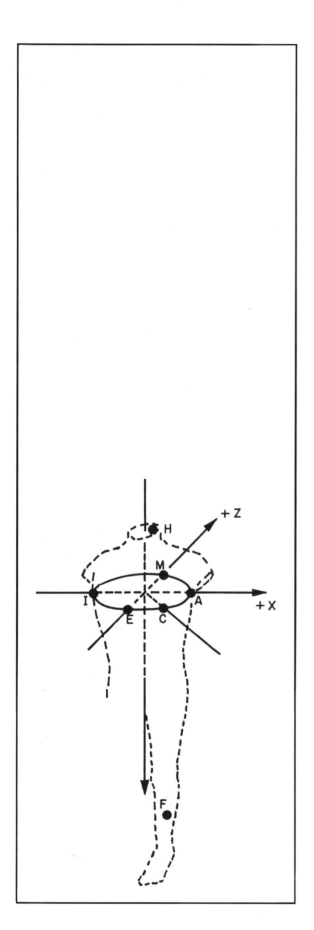

Distributed in Great Britain by Blackwell Scientific Publications, Oxford and Edinburgh

Library of Congress Catalog Card Number 70−143330

Printed in the United States of America

1   3   5   4   2

Preface

Vectorcardiography is a relatively recent medical development which represents a scientific approach to recording and interpreting electrical events of the heart. This approach has gained a widespread recognition as being imperative for a sound understanding of "conventional" electrocardiography as well as being a new tool facilitating the diagnosis of heart disease.

The spread of recognition has not, however, been synonymous with the spread of understanding of the fundamentals of vectorcardiography. Even in the academic world, and to a much greater extent outside it, the spread of understanding has been confined to a relatively small group of experts. This condition is unfortunate, in the sense that it greatly limits the use of this valuable technique in medical research and practice.

The difficulty in understanding of vectorcardiography stems from the fact that it employs quite a few biophysical and mathematical concepts the use of which has been neglected in medical education. The problem is aggravated by the lack of a simple and yet sufficiently comprehensive textbook on vectorcardiography.

This book has been written to provide a rational, systematic presentation of the fundamentals underlying vectorcardiography and to familiarize the medical man with the essential features of vectorcardiographic patterns encountered in various clinical conditions of the heart. This presentation is not at all conventional, departing sharply from tradition both in subject matter and in approach.

Another feature worthy of explicit statement is the use of a large number of drawings to stimulate the imagination in forming a geometric image of electrical events in the heart. It is hoped that this book will help to develop this important sense.

To illustrate typical vectorcardiographic patterns more clearly and thoroughly it was decided to use diagrammatic illustrations rather than photographs of the original tracings. This decision is considered justified since such diagrams are more suitable to demonstrating the criteria by which VCG patterns can be classified into different diagnostic categories. This is not the case with photographs of VCG tracings which represent unique patterns and thus do not lend themselves easily to any generalization.

Each illustration has been set in a wide margin apart from the main text and has been given the number of the part in which it appears followed by a hyphen and a serial number; thus (Fig. 3-8) means in Part 3 Figure 8.

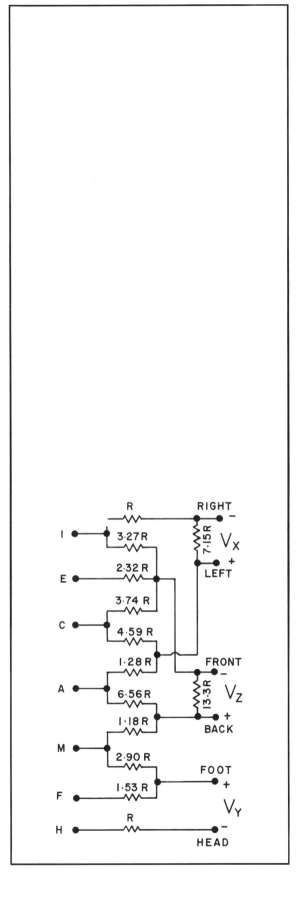

Acknowledgments

As must be true of anyone writing a textbook, the debts I owe are many: to my colleagues for many stimulating and helpful conversations, to my own teachers for the knowledge of, and interest in this subject, to the reviewers of early versions of the manuscript for many helpful suggestions and criticisms, and to numerous investigators in the field of vectorcardiography whose reports I have assimilated over many years of work in this field.

A very special appreciation goes to Dr. John A. Milliken who, above all others, has been essential to the origin of this book. Due to his initiative and efforts in establishing the modern vectorcardiographic laboratory at Queen's University, I have been given the opportunity to continue research and practice in vectorcardiography. A substantial portion of the material of this book has resulted from investigations supported in part by funds received from the Department of Health and Welfare of Canada and the Queen's University Trust Fund.

My appreciation extends also to Mrs. Helen Phelan for typing the manuscript, to Mr. Peter Montgomery for preparing illustrations, and to Miss Amelia Laing for assistance in assembling the bibliography.

Gratitude is expressed to Charles C Thomas Publisher for their kind permission to reproduce several illustrations from my book *Computers in Electrocardiography* and to the American Heart Association, Inc. for their permission to reproduce tables of normal values of vectorcardiographic items published by Draper *et al.*: Circulation, (*30*:853, 1964).

Finally, it is a particular pleasure to express a warm "thank you" to the J. B. Lippincott Company for their craftsmanship and helpfulness.

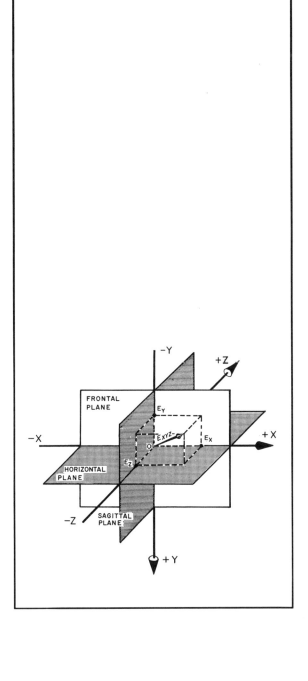

Contents

Part 1: Principles of Vectorcardiography

Electrical Activity of the Heart   2
Fundamental concepts of electricity   2
Ionic basis of the heart electricity   6
Concept of the cardiac dipole   10

Vector Representation of the Heart Electrical Forces   15
Elements of vector analysis   15
Geometry of the cardiac dipole   20

Lead Systems for Recording Electrical Activity of the Heart   29
Physical and mathematical properties of electrocardiographic leads   29
Orthogonal lead systems   33
Twelve lead system   36

Instruments Recording Electrical Activity of the Heart   40
Vectorcardiograph   40
Resolver   42
Polarcardiograph   44
Electrocardiograph   46

Methods of Analyzing Electrical Activity of the Heart   49
Reference frame for vectorcardiography   49
Analysis of X, Y, Z components   52
Analysis of vector loops   55
Analysis of the 12 lead system electrocardiograms   61

Normal Patterns of Electrical Activity of the Heart   64
Normal vectorcardiogram   64
Normal 12 lead electrocardiogram   78

Abnormal Patterns of Electrical Activity of the Heart   82
General Considerations   82
Vector interpretation of VCG abnormalities   84

Part 2: Vectorcardiogram in Cardiac Disease

Hypertrophy of the Heart Muscle   90
VCG in atrial enlargement   90
VCG in left ventricular hypertrophy   93
VCG in right ventricular hypertrophy   96
VCG in biventricular hypertrophy   102

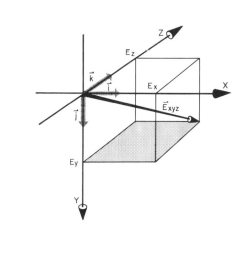

Ventricular Conduction Defects   104

  VCG in left bundle branch block   104
  VCG in right bundle branch block   107
  VCG in the Wolff-Parkinson-White syndrome   110

Myocardial Infarction, Injury and Ischemia   114

  VCG in myocardial infarction (general considera-
    tions)   114
  VCG in anterior myocardial infarction   120
  VCG in lateral myocardial infarction   122
  VCG in inferoposterior myocardial infarction   124
  VCG in strictly posterior myocardial infarction   126
  VCG in peri-infarction block   127

Miscellaneous VCG Patterns   128

  Left axis deviation   128
  Nonspecific ST-T vector changes   130
  Angina pectoris   132

Part 3: Vectorcardiogram Diagnostic Evaluation

**Differentiation Between Normal and Abnormal
  Vectorcardiograms**   137

  Logical approach to diagnosing vectorcardiograms   137
  Statistical analysis of vectorcardiograms   140
  Normal vectorcardiographic values   146
  Decision problem in evaluating vectorcardiograms   148

Interpretation of the Vectorcardiogram   154

  Vectorcardiogram reporting service   154
  Clinical value of the vectorcardiogram   157

Computer-Assisted Interpretation of VCGs   162

  Automated system for VCG data processing   162
  VCG data acquisition for computer analysis   164
  VCG waveform recognition by computer   166
  VCG diagnosis by computer   170

Part 4: Bibliography

  Principles of vectorcardiography   174
  Vectorcardiogram in cardiac disease   175
  Vectorcardiogram diagnostic evaluation   178

Index   179

Part 1
Principles of Vectorcardiography

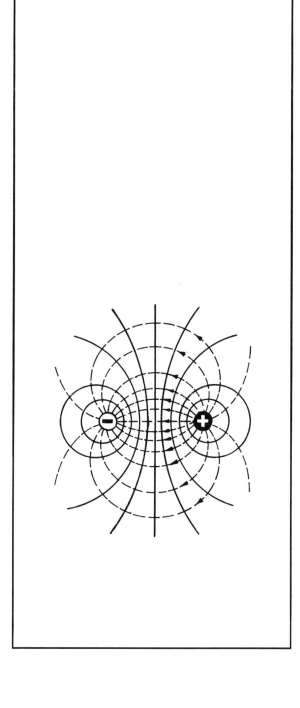

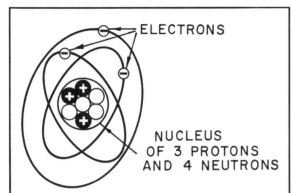

Fig. 1-1. *Symbolic picture of an atom (of lithium).*

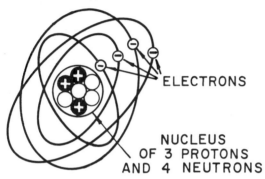

Fig. 1-2. *Symbolic picture of a negative ion (of lithium).*

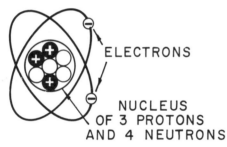

Fig. 1-3. *Symbolic picture of a positive ion (of lithium).*

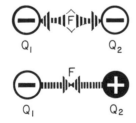

Fig. 1-4. *Schematic picture to illustrate the concept of the force of attraction (or repulsion).*

Electrical Activity of the Heart

FUNDAMENTAL CONCEPTS OF ELECTRICITY

Electric Charges

Most of the phenomena in nature have, in the last analysis, an electrical origin. This is so because all matter is composed of minute particles of negative electricity, called electrons, and small particles of positive electricity, called protons. Each ordinary atom as a whole, however, is electrically neutral, since the number of electrons is exactly matched by the number of protons (Fig. 1-1). Because only negative electricity in the form of electrons is movable, an atom can be charged either by taking away or by adding some electrons. When an electron is taken from or added to a previously neutral atom or molecule, the charged particle which is thus formed is called an "ion." If an electron is added to the atom from the outside, there is more negative than positive electricity and the atom has a "negative charge" (i.e., it becomes a negative ion, Fig. 1-2). Whereas, if an electron is taken away from the atom, there is more positive than negative electricity and the atom has a "positive charge" (i.e., it becomes a positive ion, Fig. 1-3).

Similarly-charged particles repel each other, while dissimilarly charged particles attract each other. The force of attraction (or repulsion) between two electric charges is proportional to the product of charges and is inversely proportional to the square of the distance between them (Fig. 1-4). Mathematically this law can be expressed as follows:

$$F = \frac{Q_1 Q_2}{d^2}$$

where F is the force, Q_1 and Q_2 are the charges and d is the distance between them. The unit of electrical charge is the coulomb, and it approximately amounts to 6.06×10^{18} (a million million million) electrons. A charge of one coulomb repels another equal charge of the same sign in vacuum at a distance of one meter, with a force of 9.0×10^3 newtons.

Electric Field

Whenever a body is in the neighborhood of the earth it is acted on by gravity. Such a region throughout which forces are acting is called by physicists a "field of force," and the force acting on some standard test body at any point is called the "field strength" or "field intensity" at that point. Thus, the earth is surrounded by a field of gravitational force, and the strength or intensity of the field depends on the square of the distance from the center of the earth. The test body is a mass of 1 kg., and one can say that the strength of the gravitational field at the pole is 9.83 newtons/kg., and at a height of 4,000 miles only 2.45 newtons/kg. (Fig. 1-5). In a similar way, a charged particle creates an electric field of force in its vicinity. One can visualize the field pattern by plotting lines, called lines of force, which indicate the direction of the force exerted by the field on a positive test charge.

If a test unit is placed at any point in an electrical field, the magnitude of the force which acts on it is called the electrical intensity or the strength of field. The field then has an intensity which varies inversely as the square of the distance from the center of the charge. One can visualize the field intensity by plotting lines perpendicular to the lines of force. Figure 1-6 depicts the lines of force and the lines of the field intensity for a positive charge. These lines are visualized as existing in 3-dimensional space, so that the lines of force have spherical symmetry and the lines of the field intensity become spherical surfaces. Over any given sphere about +Q the intensity of the field strength is constant in magnitude and directed radially and outward, as +Q and +1 (a test unit) repel each other. The intensity increases rapidly as the size of the sphere decreases.

Figure 1-7 depicts the lines of force and the lines of the field intensity for a negative charge. Over any given sphere about −Q the intensity of the field strength is constant in magnitude and is directed radially and toward the charge, since −Q and +1 (a test unit) attract each other. An electric field that is created around dipole (i.e., a combination of two opposite charges +Q and −Q) is discussed on page 12.

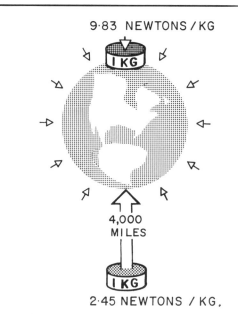

Fig. 1-5. Diagram depicting the gravitational field surrounding the earth.

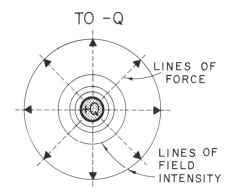

Fig. 1-6. Diagram depicting the electrical field surrounding a single positively charged particle.

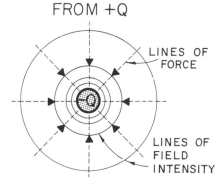

Fig. 1-7. Diagram depicting the electrical field surrounding a single negatively charged particle.

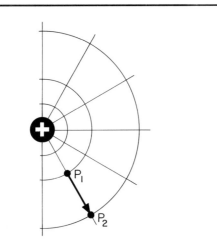

Fig. 1-8. Schematic representation of the potential difference between points P^2 and P^1 in a field of electric force.

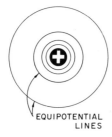

Fig. 1-9. Diagram depicting equipotential lines around a single positively charged particle.

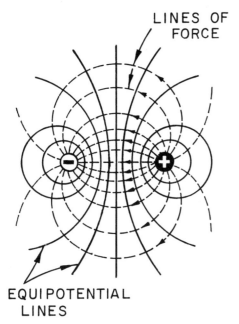

Fig. 1-10. Diagram depicting the electrical field surrounding a pair of equal positive and negative charges.

Electric Potential

Potential refers to the possibility of doing work. Any charge has the potential to do the work of moving another charge, either by attraction or repulsion. This ability of a charge to do work is its potential. When a positively charged particle is brought up toward the electric field from a distance, the motion is opposed at every point by a force Eq, where q is the charge on the particle and E is the electric intensity of the point in question, and therefore work has to be done to overcome this force. By analogy, when a man lifts a body he is moving it against the gravitational field (i.e., from a point of low gravitational potential to a point of higher gravitational potential).

The difference of electric potential between two points in a field of electric force is measured by the work done upon a test unit by the forces of field as the unit moves from one of the points to the other. A test unit or any positive charge placed in the field tends to move from a point of higher potential to a point of lower. A negative charge tends to move in the opposite direction (Fig. 1-8). The amount of work or energy necessary to move a certain number of charges from one place to another against opposition is expressed in volts. The volt is defined as the amount of work necessary to move one ampere through an opposition of 1 ohm resistance.

Since the intensity of the electric field is closely related to its potential, the lines (or surfaces) of electric intensity around the charge also represent the lines (or surfaces) of electric potential (see p. 3). Figure 1-9 shows equipotential lines around a positive charge at the center. The circles may be looked upon as cross sections of the equipotential surfaces which exist in a 3-dimensional space. Potential lines (or surfaces) are perpendicular to the lines of forces at every point in the electric field. In bringing up a positive charge to the equipotential line (or surface) a certain amount of work is required, and this work is the same, no matter to what point in the circle the unit charge is brought. This is true because in moving the unit charge along an equipotential line, no work is done.

Figure 1-10 shows the distribution of equipotential lines and lines of force which surround two equal but opposite electric charges separated by a very small distance. The lines connecting the two charges are the paths along which positive charges travel if they are left free. These lines give the directions of the field surrounding the two charges. Perpendicular to the lines of force are equipotential lines that may be regarded as different levels of energy.

Electric Current

When the potential difference between two charges forces a third charge to move, the charge in motion is an electric current. The potential difference (or voltage) can thus be visualized as a pressure that pushes charged particles (electrons or ions) in a given direction. A voltage can be present even though the charges actually are not moving, for example, in the battery of a flashlight when the switch is turned off. The battery voltage is present but the circuit is not completed, so no current can flow. This can be compared to having a pile of rocks on a platform; potential energy due to the rocks' elevation position is present even though the rocks are not moving. Once the switch is turned on, electrons stream out of the negative battery pole, through the lamp, and reenter at the positive pole (Fig. 1-11).

One may consider an electric current in a wire in much the same way as one thinks of water flowing in a pipe. Just as one speaks of water flow, in terms of gallons per second, being comprised of large numbers of molecules, one may also speak of units of electron flow. A flow of 1 coulomb per second past a cross section of conducting medium is defined as a current of 1 ampere.

Electric pressure (voltage) required to maintain the motion of charged particles is proportional to the current. In other words, if the voltage of the circuit is doubled, the current also doubles. The ratio $\dfrac{\text{voltage}}{\text{current}}$ is a constant for a given circuit and is called the "resistance." In symbol form it reads:

$$\frac{V \text{ (voltage)}}{I \text{ (current)}} = R \text{ (resistance).}$$

All materials have some resistance to current flow. Silver, copper and iron have the lowest resistivity. Other substances having relatively low resistance are carbon and solutions containing ions. Almost without exception, all other materials are insulators having resistances from thousands to millions of times that of the metals. The resistance is measured in ohms, and one says that the circuit has 1 ohm of resistance if the current is 1 ampere for a pressure of 1 volt.

The current through metals consists of a stream of electrons that drifts from the point of higher voltage to the point of lower voltage (Fig. 1-12). The current in liquids (and, consequently, in the human body) flows when ions move under the influence of potential difference existing for any reason between two parts of a liquid. Current flow in biological systems occurs in volume conductors instead of in wires. A volume conductor is a medium, such as a large vessel containing an electrolytic solution, which conducts electricity in three dimensions (Fig. 1-13).

A direct current is one in which a current always flows in one direction; an alternating current, on the other hand, flows first in one direction, then in the other. The usual lighting current is alternating current which reverses periodically 60 times each second, in a sinusoidal manner (Fig. 1-14).

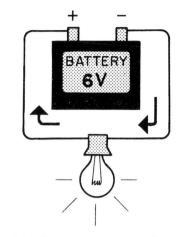

Fig. 1-11. The electric current flow in the flashlight battery.

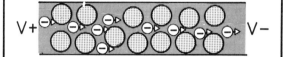

Fig. 1-12. The electric current flow in a metal (wire).

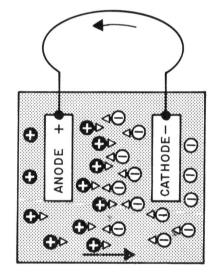

Fig. 1-13. The electric current flow in an electrolyte solution.

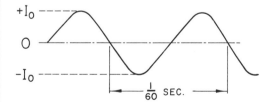

Fig. 1-14. An alternating current as represented by the sinusoidal curve.

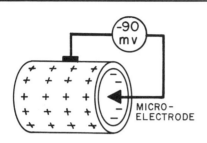

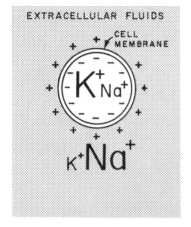

Fig. 1-15. Polarized state of a muscle fiber at rest.

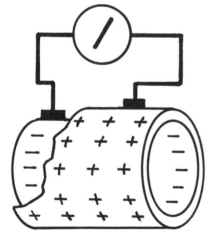

Fig. 1-16. The origin of the injury potential at the damaged cell membrane.

IONIC BASIS OF THE HEART ELECTRICITY

Resting Electrical State

The resting cardiac cell, like any other cell of excitable tissues (skeletal muscle, smooth muscle, nerve) maintains the separation of charged particles (ions) across its membrane. Positively charged particles (positive ions) are lined up along the outside of the membrane and negatively charged particles (negative ions) along the inside. A cell in this condition is said to be polarized and can be depicted diagrammatically by placing a number of plus signs along the outer side of the membrane and a similar number of minus signs along the inner side, in the manner of an electrical double layer (Fig. 1-15). Inside the cell, potassium ions predominate, outside sodium ions predominate. This condition is due to the selective ionic permeability of the cell membrane. It has been found that by inserting a microelectrode into the interior of a cardiac muscle fiber the potential of the interior of the cell is about 90 mV lower than that of the exterior. Such electronegativity of the interior of the cell with respect to the exterior is called the transmembrane potential. As long as the heart fiber is intact and is in an unactivated condition, the electrical potential difference across the cell membrane cannot be detected by measurements at the surface of the cell. It may, however, be recorded as the "injury potential" (i.e., the potential of cells with damaged cell membrane, Fig. 1-16). A "window" is thus provided into the interior of the cell. This situation occurs in an acute myocardial infarction.

Action Potential

Spontaneously, or by an external electrical stimulus, the cardiac fiber membrane becomes immediately and readily permeable to sodium ions, which therefore pass into the cell and convert its interior negative potential into a positive one; in other words, the potential of the interior of the cell exceeds that of the exterior by about 20 mV. This phenomenon is called depolarization and the potential difference occurring, due to depolarization of the cell, is called an action potential. The cell which is completely depolarized has an opposite charge distribution across its membrane (i.e., the outside of the cell is negatively charged and the inside is positively charged, Fig. 1-17). When depolarization is completed, potassium ions pass out of the cell and their efflux continues until the action potential is annihilated. This process is called repolarization (Fig. 1-18).

In order to maintain the normal concentration gradients for these ions, an active transport system (so-called sodium pump) must extrude the excess of sodium ions which entered during depolarization and pump in an equivalent amount of potassium ions which passed out during repolarization (Fig. 1-19).

During the course of activation, the area of increased membrane permeability (with associated action potential) travels rapidly along the heart muscle fiber. This movement produces a flow of electrical current and changes in potential, which can be recorded from the surface of the intact cell. The potential difference measured by the galvanometer arises because negative (depolarized) and positive (polarized) areas act effectively as a current dipole (i.e., a physical combination of two equal but opposite in sign charges that exert a certain force on each other). This concept is described in greater detail on page 12.

In conclusion, myocardial cells produce no external potentials as long as they are either completely polarized or completely depolarized. Potentials are recorded only from a transition zone between the polarized and depolarized regions, which attract each other with a certain force and thus set up an infinitesimal electric field.

In thinking about the activation process, it is convenient to regard the transitional zone as a cross-sectional disc that separates surface elements in the resting state from those in the activated state and moves along the fiber from the activated end toward the unactivated end (Fig. 1-20). Each pair of two opposite charges across the disc form an infinitesimal dipole, which subsequently can be depicted by an arrow (vector) pointing toward the positive (or resting) portion of the cell surface. By summing up these dipoles (vectors), the resultant dipole (vector) is obtained, which represents the total electrical activity of the fiber (Fig. 1-21).

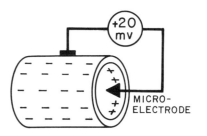

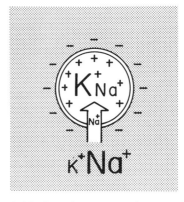

Fig. 1-17. Depolarization of a muscle fiber due to an influx of sodium ions from the extracellular fluid.

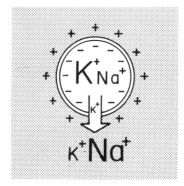

Fig. 1-18. Repolarization of a muscle fiber due to an efflux of potassium ions.

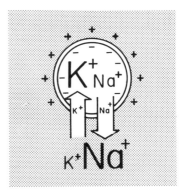

Fig. 1-19. Restoration of ionic balance.

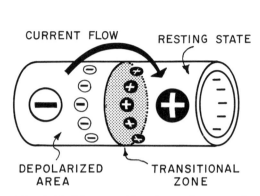

Fig. 1-20. The transitional zone between the activated and inactivated areas on the surface of a myocardial fiber as a site of microscopic dipoles.

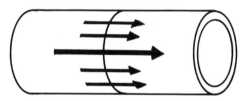

Fig. 1-21. Vectors representing individual dipoles and the resultant vector yielded by summing the individual dipole vectors.

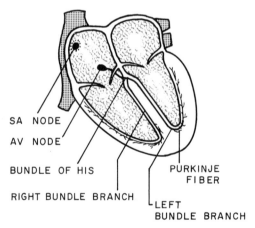

Fig. 1-22. Diagram depicting the specialized conduction system of the heart.

Spread and Regression of Activation

Activation of the heart muscle is propagated at a very rapid rate and in an orderly manner. The process of the depolarization of the heart muscle originates in the sino-atrial (SA) node, which is situated in the wall of the right auricle near the entrance of the superior vena cava. The cells of the SA node demonstrate a spontaneous depolarization which occurs 60-100 times a minute in a rhythmic fashion. Because of this capability, the SA node is designated as a pacemaker. However, all areas of the heart muscle have the potential ability to serve in this capacity (an inherent property of the cardiac tissue), but they assume this role only under abnormal circumstances. From the sino-atrial node, the process of depolarization spreads radially throughout the atria along ordinary atrial myocardial fibers and is taken over by the atrioventricular (AV) node, which is located near the top of the ventricular septum. Here, after depolarization of the atria, a physiological delay in the conduction takes place resulting in a brief electrical "silence." The AV node in turn activates the bundle of His which divides into two branches serving the right and left ventricles. Through these branches the stimulus finally passes to the Purkinje's fibers, which directly activate the innermost layer of the myocardium (Fig. 1-22).

The first part of the ventricles to be activated is the left endocardial surface of the midportion of the septum, then the impulse spreads to the right anterior and right posterior ventricles. The apex and left posterior ventricle is excited later and finally the upper septum and the high, posterior wall of the right and left ventricles (collectively termed the base of the heart) are activated. Depolarization proceeds from the inner surface of the ventricular walls toward the outer surface through the ventricular muscle. Each stage of depolarization of the ventricles can be represented by an equivalent dipole which consequently may be depicted by a vector. The spread of depolarization of the ventricles is illustrated by the light portion of the ventricle in Figure 1-23, and the equivalent dipole for each stage of depolarization can be represented by a vector as shown in Figure 1-24.

Once heart muscle becomes depolarized, approximately 0.1 second elapses before repolarization begins. Repolarization takes place more slowly than depolarization and occurs in the opposite direction, namely from the epicardium to the endocardium. Thus, the vectors representing repolarization are expected to be oriented in the opposite direction from the depolarization vectors. This state is found only in the case of atrial repolarization. However, the repolarization vectors of the ventricles are oriented in the same direction as the depolarization vectors. The discrepancy between the observed and the expected orientation of the repolarization vectors has been accounted for by pressure and temperature gradients between the endocardium and myocardium and by disorders of myocardial metabolism, but the definite factors are still uncertain.

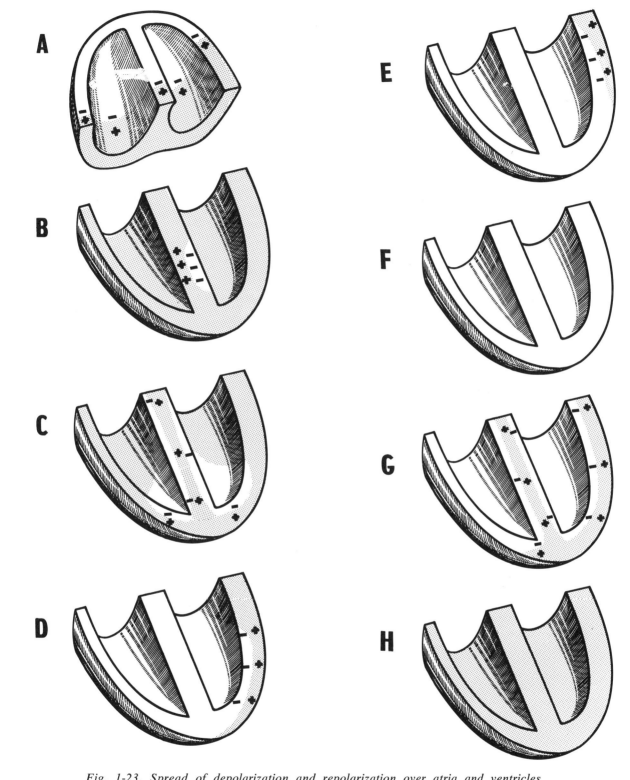

Fig. 1-23. Spread of depolarization and repolarization over atria and ventricles.
A) Atrial depolarization; B) septal depolarization; C) apical depolarization; D) left
ventricular depolarization; E) basal depolarization; F) complete depolarization; G)
ventricular repolarization; H) complete repolarization.

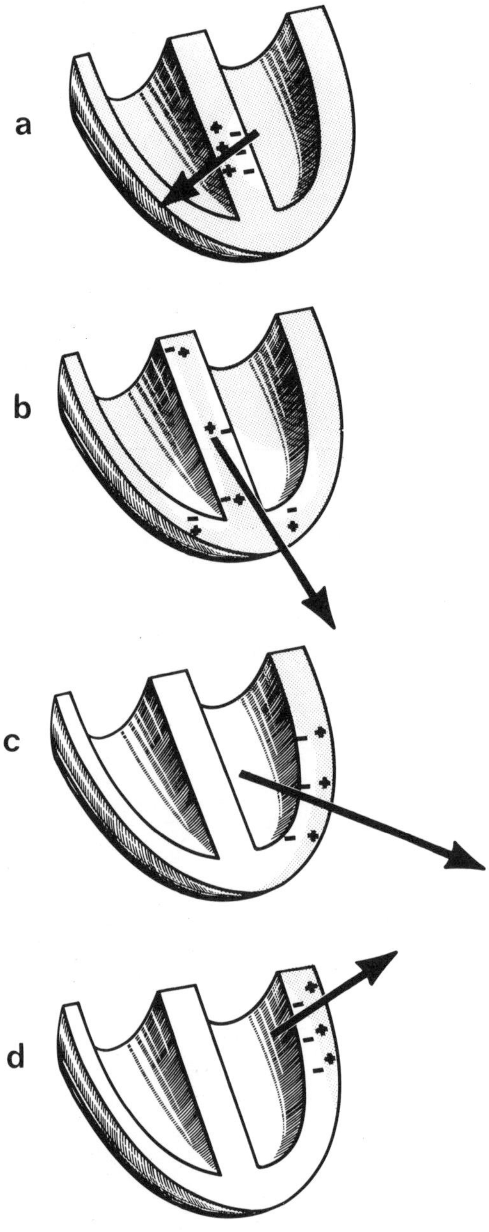

Fig. 1-24. Depolarization of the ventricles as represented by equivalent dipole for each stage.

CONCEPT OF THE CARDIAC DIPOLE

Origin of the Cardiac Dipole

It has been explained previously that all of the point sources of activity in a single fiber summate. Further aggregation of the effects of each and all of the fibers results in a total electrical effect for the whole heart, which may be assumed to originate from a single dipole. Thus, it is permissible to regard this dipole as the equivalent cardiac generator, or simply the cardiac dipole.

It is assumed that during the cardiac cycle the equivalent dipole remains at a fixed location but that its magnitude and orientation change from instant to instant. Therefore it becomes legitimate, and convenient, to study the changing pattern of distribution of potentials at the body surface in terms of changing magnitude and orientation of the equivalent dipole.

The processes of depolarization and repolarization can be broken into many time intervals and each can be represented by a resultant dipole or vector. These vectors can be considered to be directed from endocardium to epicardium. Strictly speaking, this is not true in the case of atrial repolarization, which spreads from epicardium to endocardium, but those vectors are very small and practically of no diagnostic significance.

As an example, let us consider the ventricular depolarization process. When one region of the heart becomes electronegative (depolarized) it acts as a dipole to the remainder. If all parts of the heart depolarized and repolarized simultaneously, there would be no way of detecting the electrical activity from a distant point as is done in vectorcardiography. Thus, recording electrical activity of the heart from the body surface is possible only due to asynchrony of depolarization of different parts of the heart.

On the basis of the experimental data, the ventricular depolarization process can be broken down into the following resultant, instant-to-instant cardiac dipoles (or vectors) as shown in Figure 1-24.

1. The 0.01 second septal vector represents depolarization of the left endocardial surface of the middle part of the septum; this vector is directed anteriorly, to the right and somewhat superiorly or inferiorly.

2. The 0.02 second apicoanterior vector represents depolarization of the lower portion of the septum and apicoanterior wall of the right and left ventricle; this vector is directed anteriorly, to the left and inferiorly.

3. The 0.04 second left ventricular vector represents depolarization of the lateral wall of the right ventricle and the free wall of the left ventricle; because electrical forces of the left ventricle dominate completely the small right ventricular forces, the 0.04 second vector is almost identical with its left ventricular component; this vector is directed to the left, posteriorly, and slightly inferiorly.

4. The 0.06 second terminal, or basal vector represents depolarization of the posterolateral and basal wall of the left ventricle, basal portion of the septum and the base of right ventricle; this vector is directed to the left, superiorly, and posteriorly.

Thus, depolarization of the ventricles is a series of single instantaneous vectors of successively changing magnitude and direction during the heart cycle. It is obvious that the resultant vector at a given instant is oriented in a three-dimensional space, but for simplicity only the frontal plane projections of the spatial vectors are shown in Figure 1-24.

Some studies have demonstrated that a single dipole is not an adequate equivalent generator, especially in the case of abnormal subjects. Multiple dipoles and multipoles have been proposed as alternative models to account more adequately for a complex pattern of potential distribution recorded at the body surface. However, the clinical importance of such nondipolar information has not yet been sufficiently examined.

Physics of the Cardiac Dipole

The cardiac dipole is like a pair of two concentrated charges of equal magnitude but of opposite polarity—one positive (a source), the other negative (a sink)—separated by an infinitesimally small distance (Fig. 1-25). For comparison, the terminals of a battery also constitute a dipole. The product of the magnitude of either charge and the displacement between them is called the dipole moment and represents the strength of the dipole.

Since the displacement between the sink and the source is vanishingly small, the magnitude of either charge predominantly accounts for the strength of the dipole. To completely specify the dipole, it is also necessary to consider its direction, which is defined as the line from the sink to the source. Because the dipole has both magnitude and direction it can be represented by a vector (see page 12). The length of this vector is proportional to the dipole magnitude; the direction is parallel to the dipole axis and is oriented from the negative charge to the positive charge (Fig. 1-26).

When a dipole is placed in a conductive medium (for example, an electrolyte solution) a current is set up throughout the whole medium; a medium of this kind is called a volume conductor. In a conductor in which a current is flowing, different points, in general, are at different potentials. The lines comprised of points of equal potential, or isopotential lines, form, in comparison, a series of curves which intersect at a right angle the lines of current flow. The latter flow from the positive to the negative pole, according to the usual convention (see page 12).

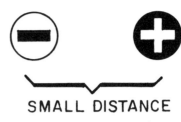

SMALL DISTANCE

Fig. 1-25. Two charges +Q and −Q a small distance apart constitute a dipole.

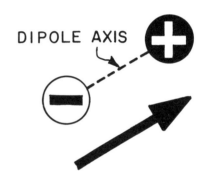

DIPOLE AXIS

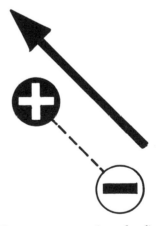

Fig. 1-26. Vector representation of a dipole.

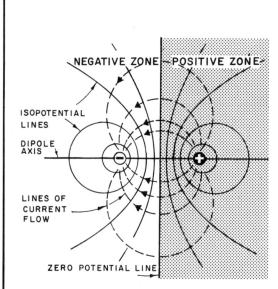

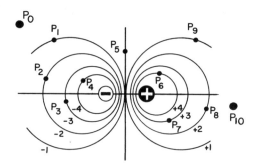

Fig. 1-27. A 2-dimensional pattern of the current field generated by a single dipole.

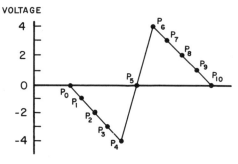

Fig. 1-28. Recording of potential differences within the electrical field surrounding a hypothetical dipole with the positive pole of +5V and the negative pole of −5V.

In Figure 1-27, the pattern is shown of a planar section through the current field which is generated by a dipole in a homogeneous, isotropic and infinitely large volume conductor. A three-dimensional idea of the current flow pattern is obtained by rotating the figure about the axis of the dipole; the equipotential lines then become equipotential planes, enclosing one another as successive shells. The line passing through the poles is defined as the axis of the dipole. The line perpendicular to the dipole axis at the halfway point between the two poles is the zero potential line and is an excellent reference point for the measurement of potential anywhere in the medium. Theoretically, the zero potential line is at electrical infinity. In practice one may approach it by placing one (negative) electrode of the galvanometer remotely from the dipole, or by averaging potential differences over the body surface. Between any 2 points within a volume conductor, one can measure the algebraic difference between their potentials.

Figure 1-28 illustrates the recording of the potential difference between various points in the electrical field surrounding a hypothetical dipole with the positive pole of +5V and the negative pole of −5V. One (negative) electrode of the galvanometer is placed at point P_0 remote from the dipole; another (positive) electrode is placed at different points and the voltage at each point is plotted on a voltage scale. If the negative electrode were placed at point P_2 and the positive one were at point P_6 the resulting voltage would be 2 volts.

Electrical Field Surrounding the Cardiac Dipole

The human body, by virtue of the chemical nature of its tissue fluids, is essentially a volume conductor (i.e., a medium that permits the conduction of electricity in three dimensions), with the boundary being limited by the body surface. Thus, when the current dipole originates in the heart it sets up an electrical field at the body surface, and potential variations within this field are easily measured.

In a volume conductor, the paths taken by the current depend upon the structure and geometry of the volume conductor. When the volume conductor is homogeneous, isotropic, infinitely large (in comparison to the dipole) and the dipole is located centrally, then the distribution of currents and potentials is symmetrical and obeys the simple law for the voltage induced at a distant point by a dipole.

According to this law, the electrical potential at any point P in a volume conductor is

$$V_P = \mu \cos \theta / d^2$$

where μ is the dipole moment (equal to the product of the charge and the length of the dipole), d is the distance from the point P to the center of the dipole, and θ is the angle between the dipole axis and the line to that distant point P (Fig. 1-29). Thus the potential varies inversely with the square of the distance and is dependent upon the angle that the line from the dipole to the point P makes with respect to the axis of the dipole.

To illustrate the way these factors influence the potentials recorded at various points in the electrical field, let us examine Figure 1-30. Proceeding to the right from the positive pole, the potential progressively diminishes. If at P_1 the potential is found to be +4V, then at P_2, which is exactly twice as far as P_1 from the center of the dipole, the potential is +1V. If point P_3 is the same distance as point P_1 from the center of the dipole but the line connecting P_3 and the center intersects the dipole axis at an angle of 60 degrees, then the potential at P_3 is found to be +4 cos 60° = +2V. If the strength of the dipole is doubled then the potential at P_1 becomes +8V.

The above discussed relationship between the dipole at the potential at a distant point applies only for a dipole immersed in a homogeneous, isotropic and infinitely large volume conductor. The human body, however, is an inhomogeneous, anisotropic, finite-sized and irregular-shaped volume conductor and the heart dipole is located eccentrically. But, in practice this inhomogeneity seems to be rather unimportant except perhaps for the low resistance and consequent short-circuiting effect of blood within the heart cavities. That short-circuiting effect of blood within the heart presumably diminishes the effect of all the separate sources and leads to a unification of electrical activity, which lends further support to the hypothesis that the heart behaves as a single dipole. However, other factors, especially a finite-sized and irregular-shaped volume conductor and an eccentrically located dipole are responsible for the fact that the heart dipole currents spread in a complex topographical fashion; and characteristics of the human body as a volume conductor can be anticipated by actual trial on living human subjects, or by studying models, rather than from theoretical speculations and purely mathematical calculations.

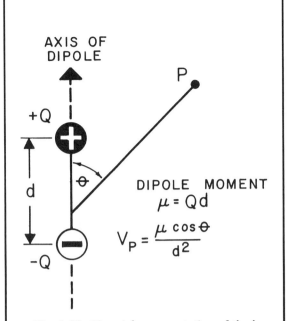

Fig. 1-29. *Pictorial representation of the law governing the voltage induced by a dipole at a distant point P.*

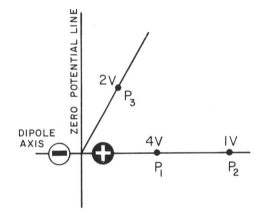

Fig. 1-30. *Example illustrating the law governing the voltage induced by a dipole.*

Vector Representation of the Heart Electrical Forces

ELEMENTS OF VECTOR ANALYSIS

Definition of a Vector

The study of an electrical activity of the heart in terms of dipole generators can be given a powerful additional significance through the use of a vectorial treatment. This approach makes the biophysical concept of the heart dipole more tangible and easier to grasp.

Before introducing elements of vector analysis essential to vectorcardiography, the clear distinction between scalar and vector quantities is necessary. Quantities, such as the number of inhabitants of a city, or the mass of a body, or the temperature which can be completely specified by a number are called scalars (or scalar quantities). On the other hand, quantities such as a displacement, or a velocity, or an acceleration, or the electric intensity, or the dipole axis, require a specification of the direction as well as magnitude for their complete identification and are called vectors (or vector quantities).

A vector can be represented graphically by a directed line segment (i.e., an arrow with an arrowhead indicating its direction and the length of the line indicating its magnitude). The point at which the directed line begins is called the origin of the vector; the point at which the directed line ends is called the terminus of the vector (Fig. 1-31).

In text, a vector is represented by a single letter written in boldface, such as **A** or **a**. Boldface type is, however, impracticable to reproduce on paper and, therefore, it is recommended that a vector quantity be designated by a symbol with an arrow or a bar above it, such as $\vec{A}$ or $\overline{A}$. The magnitude or length of the vector is denoted by a letter and symbol within brackets, such as $|\vec{A}|$. This signifies the absolute value of A (i.e., the non-negative one of the numbers A and $-$A); for example, $|5| = 5$, $|-7| = 7$. A vector also may be represented by a pair of capital letters, the first referring to the origin and the last referring to the end of the vector (Fig. 1-31).

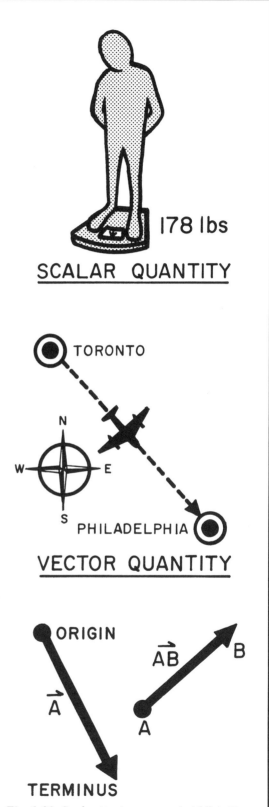

Fig. 1-31. Scalar (top) vs vector (middle). Geometrical representation of a vector (bottom).

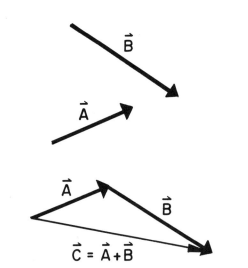

Fig. 1-32. The origin-to-terminus method of adding 2 vectors.

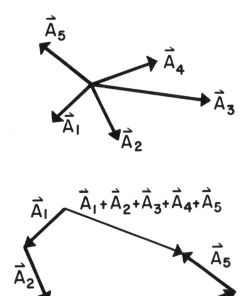

Fig. 1-33. The origin-to-terminus method of adding 5 vectors having a common origin.

Addition and Subtraction of Vectors

In the study of the heart electrical activity it is frequently useful—and often necessary—to represent the sum of two or more vectors by a resultant vector. This sum can be determined by means of two methods.

One method of calculating the sum of vectors is known as the origin-to-terminus method. In this method the sum or resultant of vectors $\vec{A}$ and $\vec{B}$ is a vector $\vec{C}$, formed by placing the initial point of vector $\vec{B}$ on the terminal point of vector $\vec{A}$ and joining the initial point of $\vec{A}$ to the terminal point of $\vec{B}$ (Fig. 1-32). This definition of addition can be extended to find the sum of n vectors $\vec{A}_1$, $\vec{A}_2$ . . . $\vec{A}_n$, of course. The geometric process may be described simply as follows: Move $\vec{A}_2$ so that its origin is at the terminus of $\vec{A}_1$; move $\vec{A}_3$ so that its origin is at the terminus of $\vec{A}_2$; continue this process until $\vec{A}_n$ is placed with its origin at the terminus of $\vec{A}_{n-1}$. The sum of vectors $\vec{A}_1$, $\vec{A}_2$, $\vec{A}_3$ . . . $\vec{A}_n$ is then the vector whose origin coincides with the origin of $\vec{A}_1$ and whose terminus coincides with the terminus of $\vec{A}_n$. Figure 1-33 shows how five vectors can be added in this way.

When only two vectors are to be added, the so-called parallelogram law is used. This method consists of the following steps:

1. If necessary, move one vector (without changing its direction) until both vectors have the same initial point.

2. Draw the parallelogram determined by vectors.

3. Take the directed diagonal that has the same initial point as vectors.

Figure 1-34 shows how two vectors $\vec{A}$ and $\vec{B}$ are added using the parallelogram law. Three vectors can be added by summing up two vectors and then adding the third vector to the sum of the other two (Fig. 1-35). In a similar way, one can add any number of vectors.

A vector is subtracted by reversing its direction and then adding it. Placing a negative sign in front of the vector $\vec{A}$ indicates that the vector $-\vec{A}$ has a direction 180° from that of the vector $\vec{A}$; however, the magnitude of the vector $-\vec{A}$ is equal to $\vec{A}$. To subtract vector $\vec{B}$ from vector $\vec{A}$, one has to reverse the direction of vector $\vec{B}$, then translate the origins of the two vectors to a common origin, complete the parallelogram of which the vectors form two sides and finally draw the diagonal from the origin of the two vectors (Fig. 1-36).

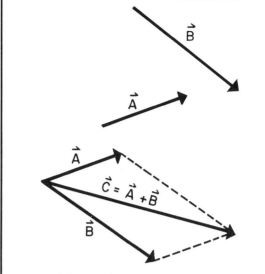

Fig. 1-34. Method of adding 2 vectors by means of the parallelogram law.

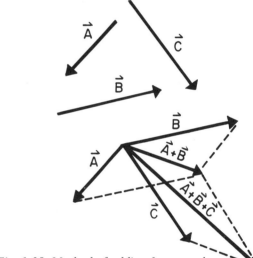

Fig. 1-35. Method of adding 3 vectors by means of the parallelogram law.

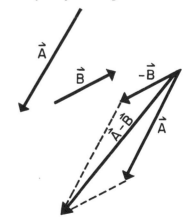

Fig. 1-36. Method of subtracting vectors by reversing the direction of the vector being subtracted and then adding it.

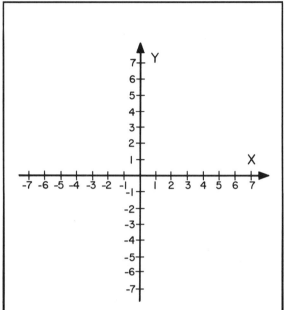

Fig. 1-37. The Cartesian coordinate system in a plane.

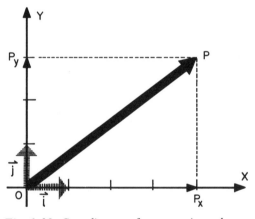

Fig. 1-38. Coordinates of a vector in a plane.

Decomposition of a Vector

By reversing the process of addition, any vector may be decomposed into two or more vectors in any arbitrary direction, as long as the sum of the component vectors equals the original vector. The most useful decomposition of a vector into component vectors is along orthogonal axes of the Cartesian coordinate system.

The Cartesian coordinate system in a plane is obtained by drawing two perpendicular straight lines, one horizontal and one vertical; the horizontal line is called the X axis or axis of abscissa, while the vertical line is called the Y axis or axis of ordinates. The point of intersection of these two axes is labeled O and is called the origin. The positive direction is upward on the Y axis and to the right on the X axis. On the X and Y axes scales are marked off with equal unit distances using the same unit of length on both axes (Fig. 1-37).

Now consider any vector $\overrightarrow{OP}$ in the plane originating at O. From the end point P drop perpendiculars to the X and Y axes. Call P_x and P_y the feet of these perpendiculars on the X and Y axes, respectively. The real number associated with P_x on the X axis is called the X coordinate (or abscissa) of P and the real number associated with P_y on the Y axis is called the Y coordinate (or ordinate) of P.

To express vector $\overrightarrow{OP}$ as the sum of two vectors parallel to coordinate axes X and Y, lay a unit vector (i.e., a vector which has the magnitude of 1) along each coordinate axis as shown in Figure 1-38. Consequently, vector OP can be written in the form

$$\overrightarrow{OP} = P_x \vec{i} + P_y \vec{j}$$

where $\vec{i}$ represents the unit vector along the X axis, $\vec{j}$ represents the unit vector along the Y axis, and P_x and P_y are called the coordinates or components of OP vector on the X axis and Y axis, respectively. Thus, any vector lying on the X or Y axis can be expressed as a product of a unit vector and a scalar. For example, the vector shown in Figure 1-39 may be thought of as a unit vector multiplied by 4.

The magnitude of $\overline{OP}$ is determined from its components by using the Pythagorean theorem

$$OP^2 = P_x{}^2 + P_y{}^2$$

$$|\overrightarrow{OP}| = \sqrt{P_x{}^2 + P_y{}^2}.$$

Following the same pattern of development as in the plane, consider any vector OP in space. By the introduction of three mutually perpendicular axes, with the same unit of length along all three axes, the Cartesian coordinate system is obtained in a three-dimensional space (Fig. 1-40). Of course, a third line cannot be drawn through O perpendicular to X and Y axes, but a third line can be drawn through O, making an angle of roughly 135° with the X axis line and one may make believe that this line is the Z axis. From the end point P drop perpendiculars to the axes and obtain the coordinates P_x, P_y, and P_z of P. As in the above example, introduce unit vectors $\overrightarrow{i}$, $\overrightarrow{j}$, and $\overline{k}$ pointing in the direction of the positive coordinate axes. It is now clear, from previous discussion, that the vector $\overline{OP}$ can be decomposed according to the formula

$$\overrightarrow{OP} = P_x\overrightarrow{i} + P_y\overrightarrow{j} + P_z\overline{k}$$

where the numbers P_x, P_y, and P_z are the components of vector $\overrightarrow{OP}$ in the X, Y, and Z directions, respectively (Fig. 1-41).

The length of $\overrightarrow{OP}$ is calculated by successive application of the Pythagoras' theorem

$$OP^2 = OD^2 + DP^2 = OA^2 + AD^2 + DP^2 = P_x{}^2 + P_y{}^2 + P_z{}^2$$

$$|\overrightarrow{OP}| = \sqrt{P_x{}^2 + P_y{}^2 + P_z{}^2}.$$

Thus, the length of a vector is the square root of the sum of the squares of its rectangular components.

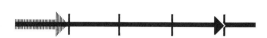

Fig. 1-39. The pictorial concept of the scalar quantity becoming a vector when multiplied by the unit vector.

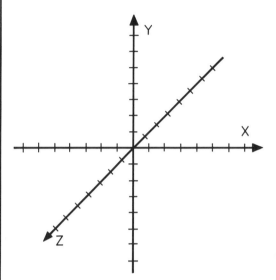

Fig. 1-40. The Cartesian coordinate system in a 3-dimensional space.

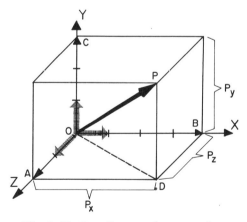

Fig. 1-41. Coordinates of a vector in a 3-dimensional space.

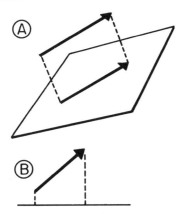

Fig. 1-42. Projection of a vector on a plane (A) and a line (B).

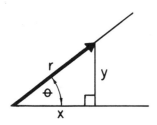

Fig. 1-43. Geometrical representation of trigonometric functions as defined with respect to the angle Θ.

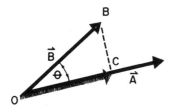

Fig. 1-44. Geometrical representation of the scalar product of 2 vectors.

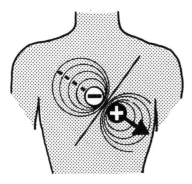

Fig. 1-45. Diagram depicting the heart vector (at a given instant) as viewed in the frontal plane.

The Scalar Product of Two Vectors

To obtain the projection of a vector onto a plane or line, it is necessary to drop 2 perpendiculars: one from the origin of the vector and another from the terminus of the vector (Fig. 1-42). Projection of a vector on a plane is a vector, whereas the projection of a vector on a line or another vector is a number. This concept is also referred to as a scalar product of 2 vectors. For a better understanding of this concept, one must be familiar with basic trigonometric elements such as a sine, cosine and tangent of an angle. These are explained with the help of Figure 1-43 and defined by the following formulas:

$$\text{sine of } \theta = \sin \theta = \frac{y}{r}$$

$$\text{cosine of } \theta = \cos \theta = \frac{x}{r}$$

$$\text{tangent of } \theta = \tan \theta = \frac{y}{x}$$

$$\text{cotangent of } \theta = \cot \theta = 1/(\tan \theta) = \frac{x}{y}$$

$$\text{cosecant of } \theta = \csc \theta = 1/(\sin \theta) = \frac{r}{y}$$

$$\text{secant of } \theta = \sec \theta = 1/(\cos \theta) = \frac{r}{x}$$

$$\sphericalangle \theta = \text{arcus tangent of } \frac{y}{x} = \text{arc tan } \frac{y}{x}$$

If $\vec{A}$ and $\vec{B}$ are any 2 vectors with common origin, then their scalar product is written as $\vec{A} \cdot \vec{B}$ (read A dot B) and defined as the product of the magnitudes of $\vec{A}$ and $\vec{B}$ and the cosine of the angle between them (Fig. 1-44). Using symbols, this is written as follows

$$\vec{A} \cdot \vec{B} = |\vec{A}| \cdot |\vec{B}| \cos \theta$$

where the symbol θ stands for the angle between $\vec{A}$ and $\vec{B}$.

The scalar product of vectors $\vec{A}$ and $\vec{B}$ can also be regarded as the projection of $\vec{B}$ on $\vec{A}$ or $\vec{A}$ on $\vec{B}$. This leads to the following geometrical interpretation of the scalar product: The scalar product of 2 vectors is the product of the length of one vector and the projection of the other upon it. By examining Figure 1-43 it becomes clear that $\overrightarrow{OB} = \vec{B}$ and OC is the projection of vector $\vec{B}$ on vector $\vec{A}$. Since OC = $|\overrightarrow{OB}| \cos \theta$, then the projection of $\vec{B}$ on $\vec{A} = |\vec{B}| \cos \theta$. Thus, it follows that the projection of one vector upon another is expressed as a scalar quantity.

GEOMETRY OF THE CARDIAC DIPOLE

Concept of the Heart Vector

The cardiac dipole, generated by the working heart, has a certain direction from − to +, and a certain magnitude (pole strength) and thus can be represented as a vector. This vector, so-called the heart vector, is oriented in the direction of the dipole axis and has magnitude proportional to the dipole moment (Fig. 1-45).

The origin of the heart vector is assumed to be in the center of the heart mass and to remain in this location throughout the single cardiac cycle. The direction and magnitude of this vector changes from moment to moment in the course of a single cardiac cycle. Consequently, for the whole cardiac cycle there are an infinite number of vectors whose terminus or arrowhead will form a continuous loop in a 3-dimensional space and this loop is called the spatial vectorcardiogram (Fig. 1-46).

Spatial vector loops cannot be completely displayed by conventional recording and only their projection on the horizontal plane (HP), sagittal plane (SP), and frontal plane (FP) can be recorded. Those projections are obtained by plotting simultaneously 2 scalar components of the heart spatial vector (i.e., XZ, YZ, and XY components). The X component is recorded along horizontal axis, the Y component is recorded along vertical axis, and the Z component is recorded along the sagittal axis (Fig. 1-47).

The spatial vectorcardiogram consists of 3 successive loops, namely: the "P loop," the "QRS loop," and the "T loop." The P loop represents the time course of all instantaneous vectors produced during atrial depolarization. The QRS loop represents the time course of all instantaneous vectors produced during ventricular depolarization. The T loop represents the time course of all instantaneous vectors produced during ventricular repolarization (Fig. 1-48). The P loop is oriented slightly to the left, inferiorly and either anteriorly or posteriorly. The main, middle part of the QRS loop tends to go inferiorly, to the left and either anteriorly or posteriorly. The direction of the initial and terminal part varies considerably with the position of the heart. The T loop has roughly the same direction as the QRS loop. All 3 loops develop from the zero point or origin. A pause occurs between the P loop and QRS loop as a result of the conduction delay in the atrioventricular node. Between the QRS loop and T loop, a similar pause takes place because both ventricles are in the fully depolarized state before repolarization sets in.

The Heart Vector Notation

A vector quantity is represented geometrically by an arrow with its direction and length related to the direction and magnitude of the quantity it describes. Throughout the text the heart vector is designated by an arrow above the letter E. In addition, it is usually necessary to put a subscript specifying the method of recording and a superscript denoting the particular heart vector. The following symbols are used:

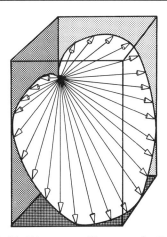

Fig. 1-46. Diagram to illustrate the formation of the spatial vector loop by the termini of an infinite number of instantaneous heart vectors.

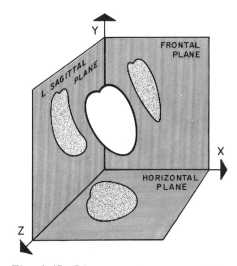

Fig. 1-47. Diagrammatic representation of the heart vector spatial loop and its planar projections. For simplicity only, the QRS loop is shown.

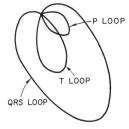

Fig. 1-48. The P, QRS, and T loops forming a normal vectorcardiogram. For simplicity only the frontal plane projection is shown.

SUPERSCRIPT / SUBSCRIPT	ATRIAL DEPOLARIZATION	VENTRICULAR DEPOLARIZATION	VENTRICULAR REPOLARIZATION
Spatial loop	$\vec{E}^{P}_{XYZ}$	$\vec{E}^{QRS}_{XYZ}$	$\vec{E}^{T}_{XYZ}$
HP loop	$\vec{E}^{P}_{XZ}$	$\vec{E}^{QRS}_{XZ}$	$\vec{E}^{T}_{XZ}$
SP loop	$\vec{E}^{P}_{YZ}$	$\vec{E}^{QRS}_{YZ}$	$\vec{E}^{T}_{YZ}$
FP loop	$\vec{E}^{P}_{XY}$	$\vec{E}^{QRS}_{XY}$	$\vec{E}^{T}_{XY}$
X component	$\vec{E}^{P}_{X}$	$\vec{E}^{QRS}_{X}$	$\vec{E}^{T}_{X}$
Y component	$\vec{E}^{P}_{Y}$	$\vec{E}^{QRS}_{Y}$	$\vec{E}^{T}_{Y}$
Z component	$\vec{E}^{P}_{Z}$	$\vec{E}^{QRS}_{Z}$	$\vec{E}^{T}_{Z}$

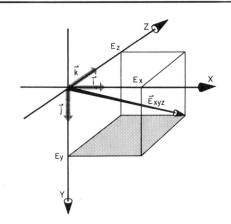

Fig. 1-49. Diagram showing the resolution of the spatial heart vector into its scalar components E_x, E_y, and E_z along the X, Y, and Z axes respectively.

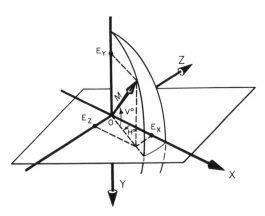

Fig. 1-50. Polar coordinate system in a 3-dimensional space. See text for details.

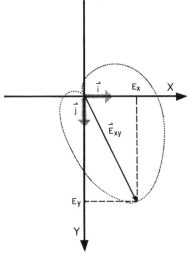

Fig. 1-51. Diagram illustrating the resolution of the frontal plane heart vector into its scalar components E_x and E_y.

In order to denote the time of the heart vector occurrence the symbol t is used. For example, the symbol $\vec{E}_{XYZ}^{QRS}$ (t) indicates that the heart vector was recorded in space during ventricular depolarization at time t, where t may be any value in the interval between the onset and the end of ventricular depolarization. The symbol $\vec{E}_{XY}^{QRS}$ (t$_{20}$) indicates that the heart vector was recorded in the frontal plane 20 milliseconds after the onset of ventricular depolarization. For identifying loops, it is convenient to use the symbol l. For example, the symbol $\vec{E}_{XZ}^{T}$ (l) indicates that the loop of ventricular repolarization was recorded in the horizontal plane.

Scalar Components of the Heart Vector

The cardiac dipole or the heart spatial vector is represented as a sum of three vectors directed along the Cartesian axes, which is provided by a special recording technique known as an orthogonal lead system. One may write:

$$\vec{E}_{XYZ} = E_X \vec{i} + E_Y \vec{j} + E_Z \vec{k}$$

where E_X, E_Y, E_Z refer to scalar components (i.e., projected magnitude) of E_{XYZ} on the orthogonal leads (coordinates) X, Y, Z, and $\vec{i}$, $\vec{j}$, and $\vec{k}$ are unit vectors directed along the X, Y, and Z axes (Fig. 1-49).

From the E_X, E_Y, and E_Z the spatial vector magnitude can be computed by:

$$|\vec{E}_{XYZ}| = \sqrt{(E_X)^2 + (E_Y)^2 + (E_Z)^2}.$$

The Cartesian coordinate system can be replaced by a polar coordinate system having the same origin and axes (Fig. 1-50). In this system, the cardiac vector is defined by three numbers:

1. The magnitude M;
2. The azimuth (i.e., the angle between the projection of the heart vector onto the horizontal plane and the left half of the X axis);
3. The elevation (i.e., the angle between the cardiac vector and the horizontal plane).

The three polar coordinates, the magnitude (M), azimuth (H°), and elevation (V°), are related to the rectangular coordinates E_X, E_Y, E_Z, by the following transformations:

$$E_X = M \cos V° \cos H°$$
$$E_Y = M \sin V°$$
$$E_Z = M \cos V° \sin H°$$

from which one can obtain the inverse relations:

$$M = \sqrt{(E_X)^2 + (E_Y)^2 + (E_Z)^2}$$

$$H° = \text{arc cos } \frac{E_X}{\sqrt{(E_Z)^2 + (E_X)^2}}$$

$$= \text{arc tan } \frac{E_Z}{E_X}$$

$$V° = \text{arc cos } \frac{\sqrt{(E_Z)^2 + (E_X)^2}}{\sqrt{(E_X)^2 + (E_Y)^2 + (E_Z)^2}}$$

$$= \text{arc tan } \frac{E_Y}{\sqrt{(E_X)^2 + (E_Z)^2}}.$$

The rectangular coordinates, as well as the polar coordinates of the heart spatial vector, are recorded as a function of time (i.e., their values are determined at various time intervals during the heart cycle). When these time intervals are very small, an approximately continuous curve is obtained. Such a curve is called a scalarcardiogram or orthogonal electrocardiogram if the rectangular coordinates of the heart vector are recorded (for details see page 33). If the polar coordinates of the heart vector are recorded, such a record is called the polarcardiogram (for details see page 45).

Plane Projection of the Heart Vector

The heart spatial vector may be described in terms of its projection upon a plane. Such a projection is obtained by vector addition of any two mutually perpendicular vectors directed along the Cartesian axes. For example, the frontal plane projection of the heart vector is the resultant vector of two vectors: one directed along X axis and another directed along Y axis (see Fig. 1-51). One may write:

$$\vec{E}_{XY} = E_X \vec{i} + E_Y \vec{j}$$

where $\vec{E}_{XY}$ stands for the projection of the spatial cardiac vector $\vec{E}_{XYZ}$ onto the frontal plane, E_X and E_Y refer to scalar components of the heart spatial vector, and $\vec{i}$ and $\vec{j}$ are unit vectors directed along the X and Y axes.

A projection of the spatial heart vector upon any plane (frontal, sagittal, horizontal) during a single cardiac cycle forms a loop-shaped figure, called a vectorcardiogram or vectorcardiogram loop. A projection of the atrial depolar cycle forms a loop-shaped figure, called a vectorcardiogram or vectorcardiogram loop. A projection of the atrial depolarization vectors forms the P loop, a projection of ventricular depolarization vectors forms the QRS loop, and a projection of ventricular repolarization vectors forms the T loop.

The magnitude and angle of the heart vector in each plane are calculated in the following way:

frontal plane $\qquad |\vec{E}_{XY}| = \sqrt{(E_X)^2 + (E_Y)^2},$
$$F° = \text{arc tan} \frac{E_Y}{E_X}$$

sagittal plane $\qquad |\vec{E}_{YZ}| = \sqrt{(E_Y)^2 + (E_Z)^2},$
$$S° = \text{arc tan} \frac{E_Y}{E_Z}$$

horizontal plane $\qquad |\vec{E}_{XZ}| = \sqrt{(E_X)^2 + (E_Z)^2},$
$$H° = \text{arc tan} \frac{E_Z}{E_X}.$$

Geometrical interpretation of the above formulas is shown in Figure 1-52.

The velocity of the inscription of the loop is expressed as a linear or angular velocity. The linear velocity in the frontal plane is calculated by the following formula:

$$V_1 = \frac{1}{\Delta t} \sqrt{(E_{X1} - E_{X2})^2 + (E_{Y1} - E_{Y2})^2}$$

where (E_{X1}, E_{X2}), (E_{Y1}, E_{Y2}) are coordinate values of two

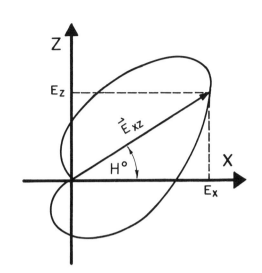

Fig. 1-52. *Geometrical interpretation of the magnitude and angle of the heart vector in a plane.*

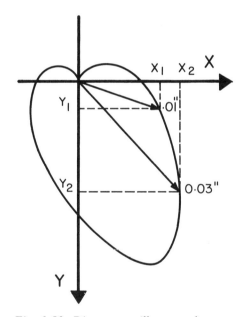

Fig. 1-53. *Diagram to illustrate the concept of a linear velocity of inscription of the VCG loop.*

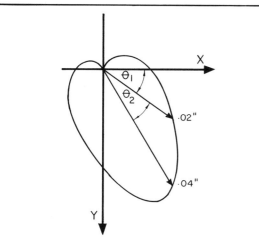

Fig. 1-54. Diagram to illustrate the concept of an angular velocity of inscription of the VCG loop.

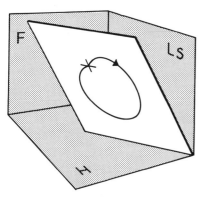

Fig. 1-55. Diagram depicting the plane of the normal QRS spatial loop.

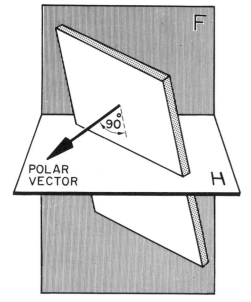

Fig. 1-56. Diagram to illustrate the concept of the polar vector (P).

successive instantaneous vectors in the frontal plane, and Δt is the time difference between these vectors (Fig. 1-53). It is possible to calculate in a similar way the linear velocity in the sagittal and horizontal planes.

The angular velocity is calculated by dividing the planar angle between two successive instantaneous vectors by the time difference between them. This is expressed by the formula:

$$V_a = \frac{\phi_2 - \phi_1}{\Delta t}$$

where ϕ_1 and ϕ_2 are azimuth angles of two successive instantaneous vectors (Fig. 1-54).

Spatial Loop of the Heart Vector

The spatial loop of the heart vector can be visualized as a continuous curve formed by the tips of a large number of momentary heart spatial vectors. Normally, such a loop lies approximately in a plane, called the "plane of predilection" (Fig. 1-55). Orientation and rotation of the spatial vectorcardiographic loop (be it the P loop, the QRS loop or the T loop) are represented by a vector perpendicular to the predilection plane (Fig. 1-56). Such a vector is called a normal vector to the plane, but in vectorcardiography it is called the "polar vector" (P).

Three rectangular coordinates X, Y, and Z of the polar vector are constituted by time integrals of the projection of the spatial QRS loop on the sagittal, horizontal and frontal planes. One may write:

$$P_X = \int_Q^S E_Y(t)dt + \int_Q^S E_Z(t)dt$$

$$P_Y = \int_Q^S E_X(t)dt + \int_Q^S E_Z(t)dt$$

$$P_Z = \int_Q^S E_X(t)dt + \int_Q^S E_Y(t)dt.$$

For convenience sake, time integrals can be approximated by calculating small triangular areas and adding them in each plane. For example, in the sagittal plane this is accomplished according to the equation:

$$P_X = \sum \Delta S \quad \text{where} \quad \Delta S = \frac{1}{2}(X_1 \cdot Z_2 - X_2 \cdot Z_1).$$

The sign of P_X, P_Y, P_Z indicates the sense of rotation of the loop in the sagittal, horizontal and frontal projections respectively; a positive sign means predominant counterclockwise rotation, and a negative sign indicates preponderance of the clockwise rotation.

The magnitude and direction of the polar vector is determined by the following formulas:

$$|\vec{P}| = \sqrt{(P_X)^2 + (P_Y)^2 + (P_Z)^2}$$

$$H° = \text{arc tan} \frac{P_Z}{P_X}$$

$$V° = \text{arc tan} \frac{P_Y}{\sqrt{(P_X)^2 + (P_Z)^2}}.$$

The planarity of the spatial QRS loop can be determined by two methods. In the first method, the mean distance from terminal points of 0.01, 0.02, 0.03, 0.06, 0.07, and 0.08 sec., to the plane of predilection is calculated (Fig. 1-57). The equation of the plane of predilection is given by:

$$AX + BY + CZ = 0$$

where X = the area of the left sagittal projection of the loop, Y = the area of the horizontal projection, Z = the area of the frontal projection, and A, B, C are coefficients. Then, the distance from the point P_i (= X_i, Y_i, Z_i) to this plane is defined by:

$$D_i = \frac{AX_i + BY_i + CZ_i}{\sqrt{X^2 + Y^2 + Z^2}}.$$

Therefore, the mean distance from the six instantaneous vectors to the plane of predilection is calculated by:

$$\text{Mean distance} = \sum_{i=1}^{6} D_i.$$

The second method is based on the calculation of three axes a, b, c of the spatial loop which is obtained through a least-square fitting procedure. The best fit of a curve inside a plane is reached when the mean square deviation between the curve and the plane is minimum. The solution of this problem yields three extreme values of the mean square deviations, the so-called eigenvalues, and, corresponding to them, eigenvectors. These eigenvectors form a new orthogonal coordinate system which is based on spatial orientation of the spatial loop. The largest eigenvalue gives an estimate of the length, the middle one of the width and the smallest one of the thickness of the loop (Fig. 1-58). The eigenvector corresponding to the smallest eigenvalue is identical to the polar vector. The ratio between the a and b axes characterizes the shape of the loop, whether it is more circular or more elongated.

The magnitude and direction of the heart vector in three-dimensional space is calculated according to the formulas on page 22. The velocity of the inscription of the spatial loop is calculated in a similar way as for the planar loop.

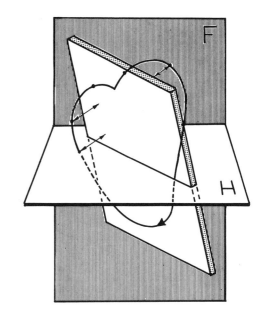

Fig. 1-57. Diagram illustrating the principle of calculating the mean distance from the 6 instantaneous heart vectors to the plane of predilection.

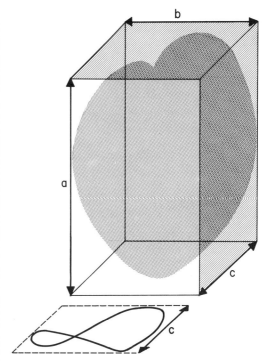

Fig. 1-58. Diagram illustrating the principle of calculating 3 axes of the spatial QRS loop.

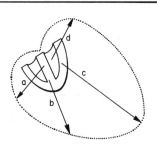

Fig. 1-59. Depolarization of the ventricles as represented by a series of instantaneous vectors. For simplicity, only 4 vectors as seen in the frontal plane are shown.

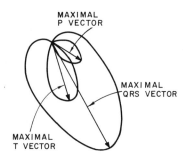

Fig. 1-60. Diagram illustrating the maximal P, QRS, and T vectors in the frontal plane.

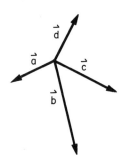

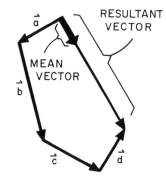

Fig. 1-61. Diagram to illustrate the difference between the mean and the resultant vector.

Instantaneous Heart Vectors

The electrical activity of the heart at any moment of a cardiac cycle is represented by a single dipole which subsequently is depicted as a vector. Such a vector is called an instantaneous heart vector. For the whole cardiac cycle there is an infinite number of instantaneous heart vectors. In Figure 1-59 only a few have been drawn for clarity.

Assume that the first region of the ventricles to undergo depolarization is the left side of the septum. The resultant dipole during this first instant is depicted by vector a in Figure 1-59. An instant later, depolarization spreads to other regions of the ventricles, and the resultant dipole at this instant has another magnitude and direction that is represented by vector b in Figure 1-59. At each subsequent instant during the cardiac cycle, with different regions of the ventricles becoming depolarized, the resultant dipole for each instant has a different magnitude and direction, as shown by the later vectors in Figure 1-59. Thus depolarization of the ventricles is depicted as if there were a series of single instantaneous vectors of successively changing magnitude and direction. A similar sequence of instantaneous vectors is generated during atrial depolarization and during ventricular repolarization.

Some instantaneous heart vectors are more important clinically than others. Of special interest in vectorcardiography are instantaneous heart vectors that have a maximal magnitude for a given part of the cardiac cycle. These are the following:

1. The instantaneous maximal P vector;
2. The instantaneous maximal QRS vector;
3. The instantaneous maximal T vector.

These vectors may be calculated along the X, Y, Z axes and/or in the frontal, horizontal, sagittal planes and/or in a three-dimensional space. Only the frontal plane projections of the maximal instantaneous heart vectors are shown in Figure 1-60.

Mean Heart Vectors

Several instantaneous vectors (i.e., vectors representing the cardiac dipole at separate moments) may be replaced by one mean, or resultant vector, which is obtained by summation of these instantaneous vectors. From the mathematical point of view there is a difference between the mean and resultant vectors in the sense that although they have the same direction, the mean vector may have different magnitude because it is obtained by dividing the sum of the n instantaneous vectors by the number n (Fig. 1-61).

The instantaneous heart vectors may be averaged over any period of time; for example, one may average instantaneous QRS vectors during the full period of ventricular depolarization, or only during a small fraction of the ventricular depolarization time. In electrocardiography the following mean vectors are usually calculated:

1. The mean P vector ($\vec{A}^P$) resulting from the instantaneous vectors of auricular depolarization (Fig. 1-62);
2. The mean QRS vector ($\vec{A}^{QRS}$) resulting from the in-

stantaneous vectors of ventricular depolarizaton (Fig. 1-62);

3. The mean T vector ($\overrightarrow{A}^T$) resulting from the instantaneous vectors of ventricular repolarization (Fig. 1-62).

In addition, the following mean vectors of the ventricular depolarization are often analyzed:

1. The septal depolarization or initial QRS vector (i.e., the vector indicating the mean direction and magnitude of the heart vectors generated within the first 10 to 15 milliseconds of ventricular depolarization, Fig. 1-63);

2. The ventricles' free walls depolarization vector, (i.e., the vector indicating the mean direction and magnitude of the heart vectors generated between the end of septal depolarization and the onset of the ventricles' base depolarization, Fig. 1-63);

3. The ventricles' base depolarization or terminal QRS vector (i.e., the vector indicating the mean direction and magnitude of the heart vectors generated during the last 10 or 15 milliseconds, Fig. 1-63).

The cardiac mean vectors provide approximate information about the magnitude and direction of electrical forces during certain periods of the cardiac cycle. Mean vectors may be calculated along the X, Y, Z axis and/or in the frontal, horizontal, sagittal planes and/or in a three-dimensional space. For simplicity, only the frontal plane projections of the mean heart vectors are shown in Figure 1-63.

To obtain, for example, the magnitude of the mean QRS vector in the X lead, one must calculate the time integral under a function representing the potential differences in the lead X plotted against time. The integral may be approximated by summing the $E_X^{QRS}(t)$ values and dividing the result by the number of E_X^{QRS} points taken. One may write:

$$|\overrightarrow{A}_X^{QRS}| = \int_Q^S E_X^{QRS}(t)dt \cong \frac{1}{n} \sum_{i=1}^{n} (E_X^{QRS})_i$$

where $\overrightarrow{A}_X^{QRS}$ stands for the mean QRS vector in lead X.

The magnitude of the mean QRS vector in the frontal plane is calculated according to the formula:

$$|\overrightarrow{A}_{XY}^{QRS}| = \sqrt{(A_X^{QRS})^2 + (A_Y^{QRS})^2}$$

where $\overrightarrow{A}_{XY}^{QRS}$ stands for the mean QRS vector in the frontal plane.

The magnitude of the mean QRS vector in three-dimensional space is calculated as follows:

$$|\overrightarrow{A}_{XYZ}^{QRS}| = \sqrt{(A_X^{QRS})^2 + (A_Y^{QRS})^2 + (A_Z^{QRS})^2}$$

where $\overrightarrow{A}_{XYZ}^{QRS}$ stands for the mean QRS vector in three-dimensional space.

The orientation of the mean vectors is calculated in a way similar to that described for instantaneous vectors.

Vectorial summation of the depolarization vectors ($\overrightarrow{A}^{QRS}$) and repolarization vectors ($\overrightarrow{A}^T$) yields a resultant vector which is called ventricular gradient in electrocardiography. It represents the net electrical effect of the differences in time course of ventricular depolarization and repolariza-

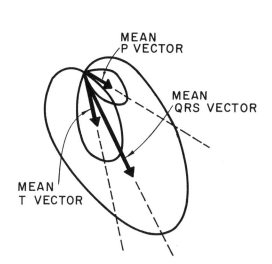

Fig. 1-62. Diagram illustrating the mean P, QRS and T vectors in the frontal plane.

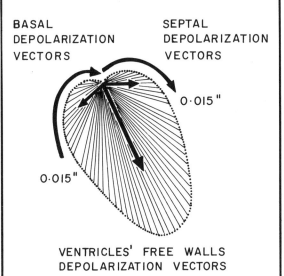

Fig. 1-63. Diagram illustrating the mean heart vectors of the ventricular depolarization in the frontal plane.

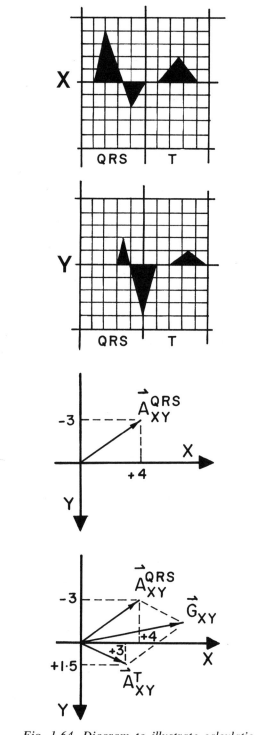

Fig. 1-64. Diagram to illustrate calculation of the ventricular gradient vector from the mean QRS and T vector (see text for details).

tion. This gradient may be determined for the X, Y, Z lead and/or for the frontal, horizontal, sagittal plane and/or in the three-dimensional space. Figure 1-64 depicts how the ventricular gradient is calculated in the frontal plane. This calculation is carried out according to the following formula:

$$\vec{A}_{XY}^{QRS} + \vec{A}_{XY}^{T} = \vec{G}_{XY}$$

where $\vec{A}_{XY}^{QRS}$ stands for the mean QRS vector in the frontal plane and $\vec{A}_{XY}^{T}$ stands for the mean T vector in the frontal plane. Here again the magnitude of the ventricular gradient in each lead, and the magnitude and the orientation of the ventricular gradient in three planes, and in space, are calculated in a way similar to that described for instantaneous and mean vectors.

Lead Systems for Recording Electrical Activity of the Heart

PHYSICAL AND MATHEMATICAL PROPERTIES OF ELECTROCARDIOGRAPHIC LEADS

Basic Requirements of Effective Leads

The cardiac dipole, as defined before, sets up an electric field which gives rise to potential differences at almost any two well-separated points on the surface of the body. Recording the potential difference between any two points on the body surface is accomplished by means of an electrode from which the current is conducted to the galvanometer of the electrocardiograph by way of the lead wire, to be returned to the body by way of a second lead wire and its electrode. This closed circuit is referred to as a lead. The term "lead" is also used to denote the vectorcardiographic or electrocardiographic record, obtained as a result of any combination of electrode placement. The lead axis is defined as an imaginary line from the negative electrode to the positive (Fig. 1-65).

From potentials manifested on the body surface, one can reconstruct the heart vector. This reconstruction is possible only by employing three leads to satisfy the following two requirements:

1. To be electrically orthogonal (i.e., their effective axes are mutually perpendicular).
2. To have equal strength (i.e., the ratio between the magnitude of the heart dipole and the amplitude of the recorded deflection are the same for all three leads).

In other words, only such a lead system, whose axes are mutually perpendicular (orthogonal) and have equal scale (or strength), can record X, Y, and Z components of the heart spatial vector at any moment during the cardiac cycle (Fig. 1-66).

Eccentricity (off-center location) of the heart dipole, variations in the anatomic location of the heart dipole from one subject to another, the finite-size and irregular-shape of the human torso, inhomogeneity of its tissues and other factors have been found to be responsible for the fact that effective axes of conventional electrocardiographic leads do not coincide with anatomical axes. Thus, the direction of a lead cannot be predicted from the site of an electrode placement. The angular discrepancies between anatomic and effective lead axes are as much as about 50° (Fig. 1-67). Also, conventional leads vary to a great extent in respect to their strength, and thus are not suitable for recording the cardiac vector (Fig. 1-68).

On the basis of theoretical assumptions and experimental results (to be discussed in the next two sections), it is found that orthogonality of lead direction and uniform strength are ensured by using appropriate resistors between the various electrodes on the body surface.

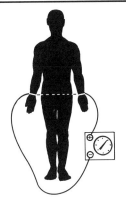

Fig. 1-65. Diagram showing the lead formed by 2 electrodes connected with the galvanometer. The dashed line represents the lead axis.

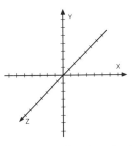

Fig. 1-66. Diagram showing the lead system whose axes are mutually perpendicular and have equal scale (strength).

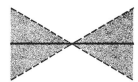

Fig. 1-67. Diagram to illustrate the discrepancy between anatomical and effective lead axis of the conventional lead L1. The shaded area indicates the range of variability in the direction of an effective lead axis of L1.

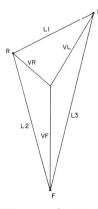

Fig. 1-68. Diagram showing the axes of the conventional limb leads in order to demonstrate their respective strength as determined from torso model studies.

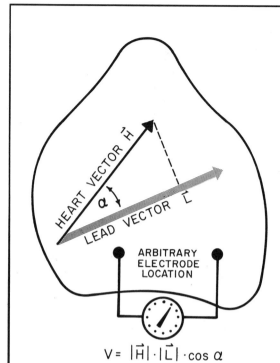

$$V = |\vec{H}| \cdot |\vec{L}| \cdot \cos \alpha$$

Fig. 1-69. Diagram illustrating the potential difference V as arising from the scalar product of the dipole vector $\vec{H}$ and the lead vector $\vec{L}$.

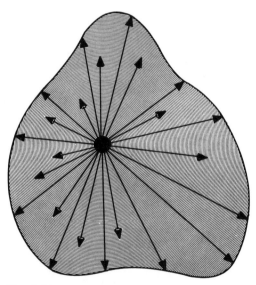

Fig. 1-70. Diagram to illustrate the concept of an image space (see text for details).

Vectorial Concept of Leads

The concept that electrical properties of a particular lead can be quantitatively described by a vector, the so-called lead vector, was suggested by Burger and van Milaan in the late forties. Such a vector has been also termed an "image vector," "lead transfer impedance," or an "effective lead axis." This vector is constant or time-invariant during the cardiac cycle. Its magnitude, or length and direction, depend upon such factors as: (1) the heart dipole location; (2) the size and shape of the human torso; (3) the inhomogeneity of tissues; (4) the location of electrodes and their relation to the cardiac dipole.

Since the conductive properties of the torso are accounted for by the lead vector, the potential difference V measured in a given lead at each instant during the cardiac cycle may be thought of as arising from the scalar (dot) product of the dipole vector $\vec{H}$ and the lead vector $\vec{L}$. Thus, the variation of the lead voltage is generated by the time-varying magnitude and direction of the heart dipole vector alone.

The scalar product of the heart vector and lead vector can be calculated by multiplying the magnitudes of these vectors by the cosine of the angle they subtend, according to the following formula:

$$V = \vec{H} \cdot \vec{L} = |\vec{H}| \cdot |\vec{L}| \cdot \cos.$$

This relation, when expressed in a different way, states that the projection of the heart dipole onto the lead vector, times its length, yields the potential difference in this lead. The potential difference recorded in a given lead (at any instant) is determined by the magnitude and direction of the heart vector, and the direction and length of the lead vector (Fig. 1-69). It also follows that the scalar product of these two vectors is largest when they are parallel and is zero when they are perpendicular.

A lead vector is commonly expressed in ohms/cm. Since this is equivalent to mV/mA − cm, and the heart dipole is expressed in mA − cm, the product of a lead vector and heart dipole is a scalar quantity expressed in millivolts (mV).

For each point on the body surface there is a corresponding lead vector. These (lead) vectors can be referred to an appropriate common origin in an image space, and their termini for all body surface points form an image surface (Fig. 1-70). There is a one-to-one correspondence between points on the body surface in real space and corresponding points on the image surface in an image space. Torso models may be used to establish the image surface, which subsequently is employed to develop leads with specially desired properties of axis orientation.

The Measurement of Lead Vectors

A number of excellent investigations have been performed during the last two decades in order to measure the direction and magnitude of lead vectors. Such investigations have been carried out on torso models shaped on the body of different subjects and filled with an electrolytic solution, (e.f. 0.1% Na Cl solution).

Using such models, artificial current dipoles of known strength can be inserted into the cardiac area of the model, and then they can be energized in three orthogonal directions X, Y, and Z, or in any other direction (Fig. 1-71). For example, when the dipole is energized in a strictly horizontal (i.e., X) direction, the potential difference recorded in a given lead can be expressed as the heart vector's X component ($\vec{H}_x$) multiplied by the vector representing this particular lead. This can be expressed by the formula

$$V_1 = \vec{H}_x \cdot \vec{L}_x.$$

In a similar fashion the potential difference produced in a given lead by the dipole oriented in the Y and Z direction can be formulated as $V_2 = \vec{H}_y \cdot \vec{L}_y$ and $V_3 = \vec{H}_z \cdot \vec{L}_z$ respectively. Then the X, Y, and Z components of a given lead vector can be easily determined because the strength of the dipole and the lead voltage are known.

Using the torso model and artificial dipoles, any number of lead vectors can be determined. Plotting these vectors from the dipole origin results in the construction of an image surface. The shape of this image surface is different from that of the anatomical body.

The magnitude and direction of a lead vector are influenced mainly by the location of a dipole within a torso model, much less by the torso shape and torso inhomogeneity. This fact is schematically illustrated in Figure 1-72, which depicts four different dipole locations, and corresponding to them, lead vectors measured in an anatomically sagittal lead. The extreme variation of the magnitude and directions of lead vectors of the four dipoles in Figure 1-72 is apparent.

It is possible to design leads which are relatively insensitive to dipole location by averaging potential differences recorded at several points rather than at the two points.

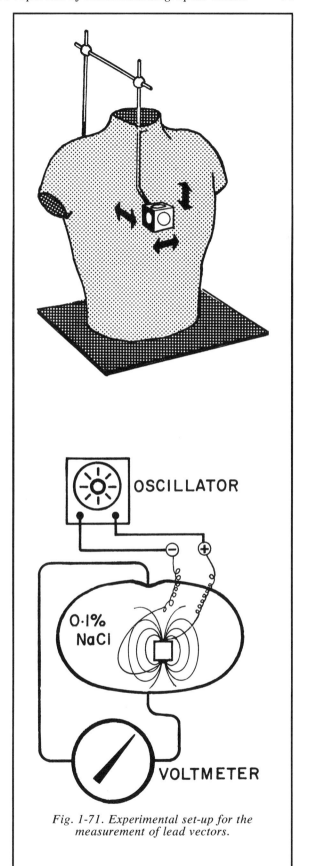

Fig. 1-71. Experimental set-up for the measurement of lead vectors.

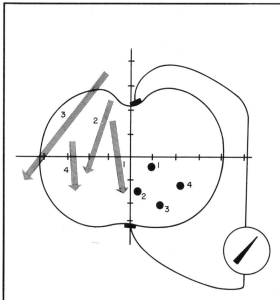

Fig. 1-72. Diagram to illustrate lead vectors as measured in an anatomically sagittal lead for 4 different dipole locations. The marked variation of the magnitude and direction of these lead vectors can be judged by referring to the X and Z axes marked in arbitrary units.

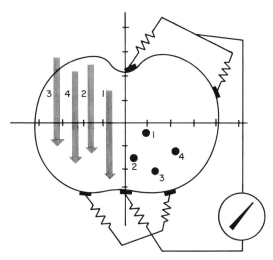

Fig. 1-73. Diagram to illustrate lead vectors as measured in an electrically sagittal lead for 4 different dipole locations. All 4 lead vectors are strictly antero-posterior and have the same magnitude.

This type of lead is shown in Figure 1-73. A combination of the anterior two electrodes forms one terminal, and a combination of the posterior two electrodes forms another terminal of the lead. The relative weighting of the contribution of each of the electrodes can be fixed by the size of the resistor interposed between each of the electrodes and the two terminals. To reduce AC interference in recording, it is preferable that the sum of the reciprocals of the resistors connected to one terminal be equivalent to the sum of the reciprocals of the resistors attached to the other terminal.

Leads which are relatively insensitive to dipole location increase the accuracy of the assumption that the equivalent heart dipole has a fixed location. Such leads are called corrected orthogonal leads; the adjective "corrected" stresses the fact that they are electrically orthogonal, thus being superior to the older vectorcardiographic leads, which were only anatomically orthogonal (see page 34).

Concerning the conventional electrocardiographic leads, their direction and strength depend critically upon the location of the heart dipole in relation to the thorax. This location differs from one subject to another and from instant to instant in the same subject.

ORTHOGONAL LEAD SYSTEMS

Orthogonal Lead System of Frank

Several corrected orthogonal lead systems have been developed in the last two decades (Frank, SVEC-III, McFee, Helm, Burger). However, only the Frank lead system has been commonly used.

This system is reasonably good as to electrical orthogonality, employs only 7 electrodes (for comparison, the SVEC-III system employs 14 electrodes) and their placement is fairly simple and is reproducible. Electrode placement in the Frank lead system is shown in Figure 1-74. Five electrodes are placed at the level of the fifth intercostal space, where the origin of the heart dipole is assumed to be. These electrodes are placed as follows:

M — on the back at the midline
E — on the front at the midline
I — right midaxillary line
A — left midaxillary line
C — between E and A (at a 45° angle).

All the points except C are relatively easy to locate. This point is usually located midway between points A and E, as measured on the surface of the chest. More accurate location requires the use of a chest protractor. The placement of the electrode at point C may offer some difficulties in obese patients with large breasts, in female subjects and patients with deformed chests. The 2 remaining electrodes are placed on the left leg (F), and on the back of the neck (H). In addition, there is a ground electrode placed on the right leg.

The electrodes are joined through resistors, as shown in Figure 1-75 to form leads, X, Y, and Z. The contribution of each electrode to the X, Y and Z leads may be expressed by the following set of equations:

$$V_X = 0.610\ V_A + 0.171\ V_C - 0.781\ V_I$$

$$V_Y = 0.655\ V_F + 0.345\ V_M - 1.000\ V_H$$

$$V_Z = 0.231\ V_C + 0.374\ V_E + 0.264\ V_I - 0.133\ V_A$$
$$- 0.736\ V_M.$$

A coefficient of 1.000 corresponds to a unit resistance, R. A unit resistance of 50,000 to 100,000 ohms is considered sufficiently high to prevent electrical errors resulting from differences in electrode skin resistance.

The choice of electrode sites and the way in which electrode potentials are combined, produce image vectors L_X, L_Y, L_Z parallel to the X, Y, and Z axes of the body, and maintain this property with good accuracy in both length and angle for a substantial range of different dipole locations and different thorax shapes. The natural lengths of image vectors L_X, L_Y, and L_Z are 174, 136, and 156 arbitrary units (often referred to as Frank units), respectively (Fig. 1-76). They are equalized to be 136 arbitrary units by means of the shunt resistors of 7.15 R and 13.3 R across the terminals of leads X and Z, respectively, as shown in Figure 1-75.

The X lead is a horizontally right-to-left lead, being left-

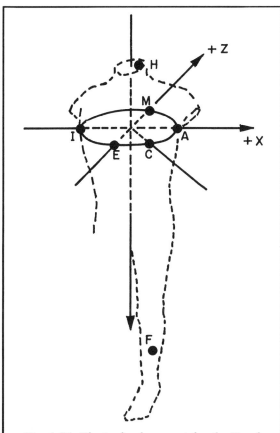

Fig. 1-74. Electrode placement for the Frank lead system.

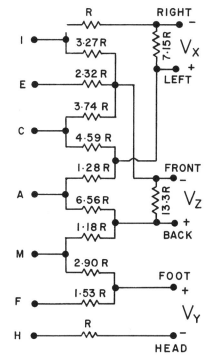

Fig. 1-75. Resistor network for the Frank lead system.

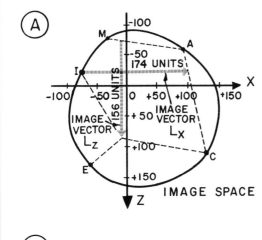

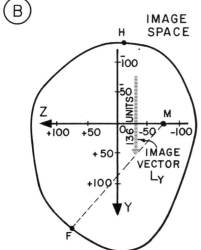

Fig. 1-76. Image vectors for the Frank's leads X, Y, and Z as they appear in the horizontal (A) and frontal (B) planes.

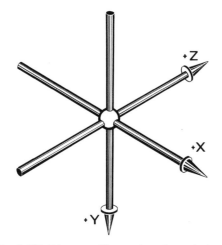

Fig. 1-77. Diagram illustrating the polarity of X, Y, and Z leads in the Frank system.

ward positive; leftward directed cardiac vectors cause an upward deflection in the X lead. The Y lead is a vertically head-to-foot lead, being footward positive; footward directed cardiac vectors cause an upward direction in the Y lead. The Z lead is a sagitally front-to-back lead, being backward positive; backward directed cardiac vectors cause an upward deflection in the Z lead (Fig. 1-77).

Uncorrected Vector Lead Systems

The first lead systems aimed at recording the heart vector did not utilize the lead vector concept. They were based on the assumption that the heart vector can be satisfactorily reconstructed, if the lead axes are orthogonal in an anatomical sense. However, model studies have revealed the rather severe inadequacies of these systems. It has been found that anatomical axes are not parallel to lead vectors; they are not mutually perpendicular or equal in length; and they are strongly dependent on dipole location.

The most popular of these uncorrected vector lead systems have been the tetrahedron and cube systems. The tetrahedron system utilizes 4 electrodes placed one each on the right arm, left arm, left leg, and on the posterior thorax just to the left of the midline, at the level of the seventh dorsal vertebra (Fig. 1-78).

The following combinations of electrodes are used to

provide three leads which are approximately anatomically perpendicular:

X lead = the left arm electrode — the right arm electrode;

Y lead = the Wilson central terminal electrode — the left leg electrode;

X lead = the Wilson central terminal electrode — the back electrode.

The cube system also utilizes 4 electrodes but they are placed on different locations: three electrodes are located one each on the left posterior axillary line, on the right posterior axillary line, and on the right anterior axillary line, all at the level of the first or second lumbar vertebra; a fourth electrode is placed on the right posterior axillary line over the scapula (Fig. 1-79).

These electrodes are arranged in the following combinations to provide X, Y, and Z leads:

X lead = the right lumbar electrode — the left lumbar electrode

Y lead = the right lumbar electrode — the right scapular electrode

Z lead = the right lumbar electrode — the right anterior electrode.

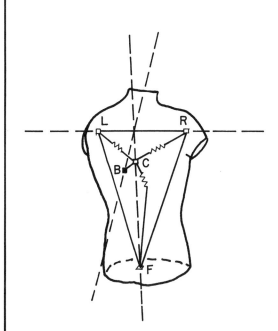

Fig. 1-78. *Electrode placement for the tetrahedron system (as viewed from the back).*

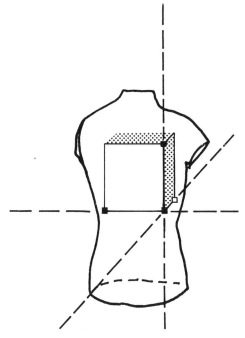

Fig. 1-79. *Electrode placement for the cube system (as viewed from the back).*

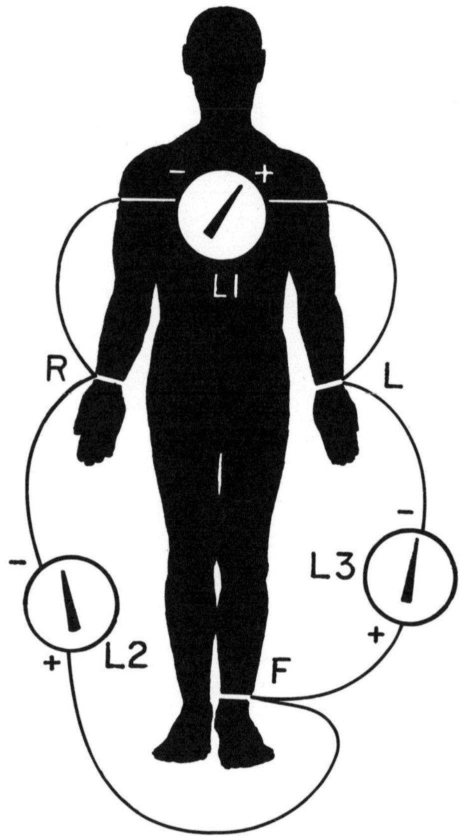

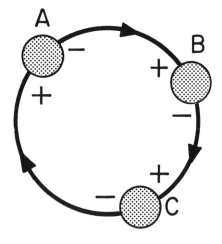

Fig. 1-80. Electrode placement for the conventional bipolar limb leads.

KIRCHHOFF'S LAW

AB + BC + CA = O

Fig. 1-81. Diagram to illustrate Kirchhoff's law.

TWELVE LEAD SYSTEM

Standard Limb Leads

The earliest system for recording potential differences between various points on the body surface was proposed by Einthoven, almost seventy years ago. This system involves three bipolar limb leads which measure the difference in potential between three pairs of electrodes placed in the following way (Fig. 1-80):

Lead L1: left arm (+) to right arm (−)
Lead L2: left leg (+) to right arm (−)
Lead L3: left leg (+) to left arm   (−).

The polarity of leads, as chosen by Einthoven, results in the recording of a positive potential difference in lead L2 in most normal cases. If Einthoven chose the polarity of lead L2 to be right arm (+) − left leg (−), then the sum of potential differences in L1, L2, and L3 would be zero. This conclusion is based on Kirchhoff's law, which states that the algebraic sum of all potential differences in a closed circuit equals zero (Fig. 1-81). Since the heart vector normally points leftward and downward, it follows that recordings in L1 and L3 are usually positive. This result implies that the recordings in L2 would have been negative to satisfy Kirchhoff's law, had Einthoven not reversed the polarity of lead L2.

To relate the electrical acitivity of the heart with potential differences recorded in these leads, Einthoven introduced the "triangle hypothesis." According to this hypothesis, the heart is considered to lie in the center of an equilateral triangle on the frontal plane of the body. The apices of this triangle (both shoulders and pubis) are regarded to be equally distant from the heart dipole and equally distant from each other. The human body is assumed to be a homogeneous and isotropic volume conductor. Since the limbs, electrically speaking, are long conductors, electrodes placed anywhere along their surface record the same potential as if they were actually placed at the apices of Einthoven's equilateral triangle (Fig. 1-82). Under these assumptions, which are only approximately valid, the potential difference recorded in any limb lead represents projection of the frontal plane heart vector on the axis of a given lead.

Since the advent of the concept of lead vectors, it has been recognized that the bipolar limb leads are not of uniform strength and therefore they can be represented more accurately by the nonequilateral triangle, the so-called Burger triangle (Fig. 1-83). This triangle is obtained by calculating image vectors for lead L1, L2, and L3 on models. When the heart vector is projected on each of the sides of the Burger triangle, the scalar voltages recorded by each lead at that instant are not equal to the magnitudes of the projections, but are equal to the product of the magnitude of the projected vector and the length of the lead. If, for example, the length of lead L2 is taken as a unity, the magnitude of the projected vector on lead L1 is reduced by a factor equal to the ratio of the length of lead L1 to the length of lead L2. Similarly, the magnitude of the projected vector on lead L3 is increased by a factor equal to the ratio of the length of lead L3 to the length of lead L2. In the case of the Einthoven equilateral triangle, the projected vector need not be multiplied by the length of any lead, since each of the three sides is considered to be of equal length.

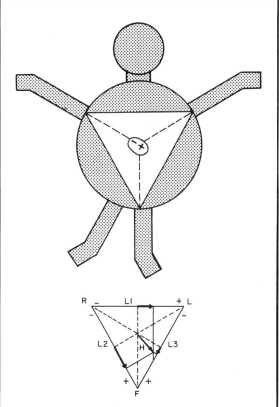

Fig. 1-82. The Einthoven equilateral triangle formed by the axes of lead L1, L2, and L3 when the body is regarded as a sphere of uniform conductivity with the heart dipole centrally located.

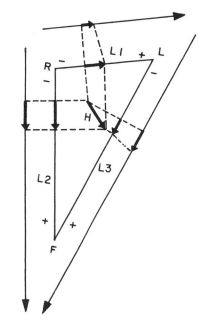

Fig. 1-83. The Burger scalene triangle demonstrating the lead vectors of the bipolar limb leads as determined from a torso model that includes spine and lungs.

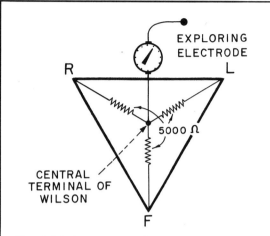

Fig. 1-84. *Diagram to illustrate a formation of the central terminal (electrode) of Wilson.*

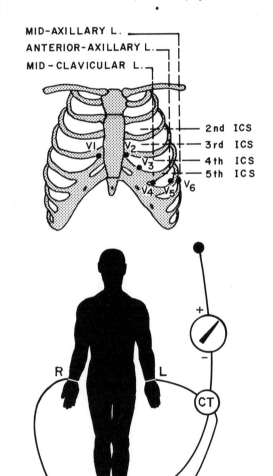

Fig. 1-85. *Positions of the exploring (chest) electrode for conventional precordial leads. CT = central terminal of Wilson.*

Unipolar Leads

In an attempt to measure the potential directly under only one electrode, rather than the potential difference between two electrodes, Wilson devised the unipolar leads. The unipolar lead consists of a negative electrode, comprising all three standard limb leads together at one point, and a positive electrode, which can be moved to a number of positions on the body surface. The negative electrode (or "central terminal") is at zero potential, since Lead L1 plus L3 plus (−) L2 equals zero (one of Kirchhoff's laws of electricity). The "central terminal" is not on the body at all, but in the electronic apparatus connected to the leads; and it is connected to each of the three standard leads by a network of resistors (usually of 5,000 ohm's resistance, Fig. 1-84).

The positive (or exploring) electrode is the active member of the pair, recording the potential variations in its immediate vicinity. The unipolar limb leads are formed by placing the exploring electrode on the right arm (VR), left arm (VL), and the left leg (VF). The unipolar precordial leads are formed by placing the exploring electrode on the chest at the following locations (Fig. 1-85):

V1 — 4th intercostal space on the right edge of sternum
V2 — 4th intercostal space on the left edge of sternum
V3 — midway between V2 and V4
V4 — 5th intercostal space in the midclavicular line
V5 — anterior axillary line at the level of V4
V6 — midaxillary line at the level of V4.

Since the deflections obtained from the unipolar limb leads were somewhat small, Goldberger devised a method of augmenting their voltage. This system, in common use on most electrocardiographs, is designated by the letter "a" or "A" (augmented) prefixed to the lead (i.e., AVR, AVL, AVF). Its end result is to increase the voltage of the unipolar limb leads by 50 percent. This result is achieved by disconnecting the central terminal from the limb to which the exploring electrode is attached (Fig. 1-86).

In the Einthoven's triangle (i.e., in the hypothetical image space), the central terminal is located at the center of gravity. Consequently, the axis of a unipolar limb lead in the Einthoven's triangle is a line joining the center of the triangle with an appropriate apex (Fig. 1-87). In summary, one may consider leads L1, L2, L3, aVR, aVL, aVF to be recordings of the X and Y components of the cardiac spatial vector (or the projection of this vector on the frontal plane) taken from different viewpoints. This can be compared with taking a series of photographs of a flag from different viewpoints around the flagpole. Lead L1 axis resembles closely the lead X axis, whereas lead aVF axis corresponds most closely to the lead Y axis.

Axes of the precordial leads lay approximately in the horizontal plane, thus recording the X and Z components of the cardiac spatial vector (or the projection of this vector on the horizontal plane) from different viewpoints. The axis of the lead V1 or V2 corresponds most closely to the lead Z axis, whereas the axis of the lead V5 or V6 responds maximally to the lead X axis (Fig. 1-88).

In effect, the 12 routine leads provide twelve views of the cardiac spatial vector. Thus, if the concept of the cardiac dipole, as a sole source of potential distribution at the body surface, is valid, then there is considerable redundancy in the standard 12 lead electrocardiogram, because the same information is obtained by recording only three orthogonal leads (X, Y, and Z).

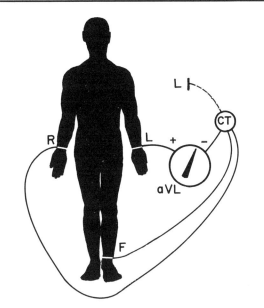

Fig. 1-86. Diagram to illustrate augmented unipolar limb leads (only aVL is shown). CT = central terminal of Wilson; the broken line indicates that the central terminal is disconnected from the left limb.

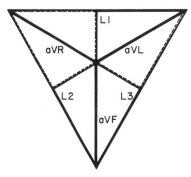

Fig. 1-87. Axes of the bipolar and unipolar limb leads in the Einthoven's triangle. The positive side of the axis is represented by a thick solid line; the negative side of the axis is represented by a broken line on top of a thin solid line.

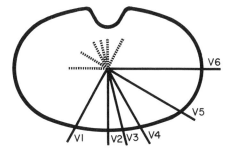

Fig. 1-88. Axes of the precordial leads as viewed in the horizontal plane. The positive side of the axis is represented by a solid line; the negative side of the axis is represented by a broken line.

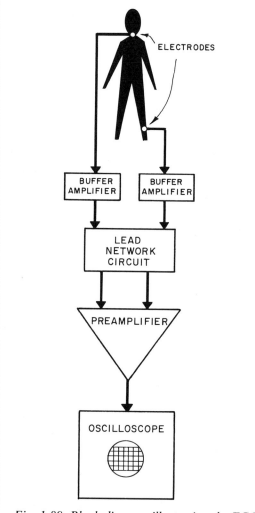

Fig. 1-89. Block diagram illustrating the ECG signal conditioning.

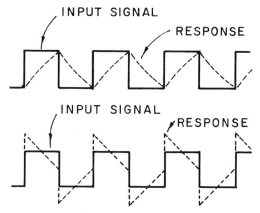

Fig. 1-90. Diagram illustrating frequency distortion of the square wave. Top: *poor high-frequency response;* bottom: *poor low-frequency response.*

Instruments Recording Electrical Activity of the Heart

VECTORCARDIOGRAPH

Signal Conditoning

The electrical signal generated by the heart and picked up by means of electrodes, is not only weak (1 to 2 millivolts), containing insufficient power in itself to activate recording devices, but frequently is accompanied by extraneous information or artifacts, detracting from or masking the desired information. Before being displayed the ECG signal undergoes a conditioning operation such as amplification, bandwidth modification or other changes necessary to make the information more usable. These operations are performed by amplifiers (Fig. 1-89).

The ECG signal represents a mixture of sinusoidal waves of different frequencies, varying both in phase and also in amplitude. The greatest portion of the ECG signal occupies a frequency range between 0.2 cps and 100 cps, but frequencies above these ranges may occur in some pathological conditions. If the measuring system is incapable of handling the higher frequency components, then sharp slopes (such as those encountred in square waves) are rounded (Fig. 1-90, top). If the system lacks low-frequency response, then the wave may be distorted, as noted in Figure 1-90, bottom.

One of the major parameters of any amplifier is the frequency response (i.e., the ability to provide a gain of the input signal through a certain range of frequencies). The lower and upper limits of an amplifier's frequency response, indicate the bandwidth at which the input signal will be satisfactorily reproduced. In more sophisticated recording devices amplifiers have adjustable frequency response controls, which enable the operator to set the lower and upper limits of frequency response at the desired level. The low frequency cutoff is usually 0.1 or 0.2 cps and the upper frequency cutoff is 60, 200 or 1000 cps.

Other important characteristics of ECG amplifiers are high input impedance and high common mode rejection. The input impedance is the ratio of voltage applied to the input to the current drawn. High input impedance is required to ensure that electrical potentials from the body surface are transferred to the amplifiers with minimum losses. In order to ensure 1 percent accuracy of voltage transferrance, the input impedance of the amplifier must be at least 100 times greater than the maximum source impedance. To reduce the effect of changes in skin impedance, a buffer amplifier is usually provided for all electrode leads (except right leg), which presents an input impedance greater than 50 megohms to the electrodes and output impedance at approximately 50 ohms to the vector lead network. Common mode rejection is the ability of an amplifier to ignore a signal that is present simultaneously at both terminals of the amplifier. This way all undesired (common) signals which could change or mask the ECG signal are rejected.

Oscilloscope Displaying

Vectorcardiograms are displayed on the face of a cathode-ray tube as it is bombarded by a moving beam of electrons. The cathode-ray tube is the basic unit of the oscilloscope. It is comprised of four parts: (a) an evacuated glass envelope, (b) an electron gun for producing a stream of electrons, (c) a means of deflecting the electron stream, and (d) a screen to transform the electrical energy of the electron beam into light.

The horizontal and vertical deflection plates vary the path of the electron beam, and a phosphor coating on the inner face of the tube emits visible light, when it is bombarded with the high-speed electrons. A voltage difference between the vertical deflection plates bends the electron beam either upward or downward, depending on the voltage polarity. The electron beam, therefore, strikes the phosphor screen at a point determined by the voltages on the deflection plates (Fig. 1-91).

When an electrocardiographic signal is applied to the oscilloscope in such a way as to deflect the electron stream in the vertical (amplitude) axis, while an internal sweep circuit deflects the stream in the horizontal axis at a regular controlled rate, scalar tracing is obtained (Fig. 1-92). When the horizontal beam sweep is turned off then the electrical signal is taken to the horizontal deflection plates and the wave form displayed is a function of the signals applied to both the vertical and horizontal axes, and the result is a two-dimensional vectorcardiogram loop (Fig. 1-93).

A frontal plane vectorcardiogram is formed using a lead representing the X coordinate as the input to the horizontal axis, and a lead representing the Y axis as the input to the vertical axis of an oscilloscope. When this is done the X input and the Y input acting simultaneously upon the beam cause the beam to be displayed in an XY plane. In a similar way, a sagittal plane and a horizontal plane vectorcardiogram are formed.

All commercial oscilloscopes employ a square wave stimulator to modulate the cathode-ray beam, which results in interruption of the loop at regular intervals, most commonly every 1, 2.5 or 5 msec. The luminous dashes are modified electronically into the form of a teardrop, the thicker end of which indicates the direction of inscription of a given loop (Fig. 1-94). The distance between the dashes indicates the speed of inscription. Closely spaced dashes signify a slow rate of inscription, widely spaced and elongated dashes a rapid speed of inscription.

These instruments also may have an automatic trigger and an adjustable delay so that only part of the cardiac cycle can be displayed on the oscilloscope. The selected portion of the VCG signal, such as the P wave, then can be presented in enlarged loop or scalar (sweep) form, while the unwanted portion of the trace is blanked out.

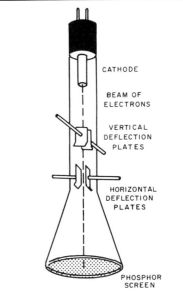

Fig. 1-91. Simplified diagram of a vectorcardiograph.

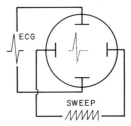

Fig. 1-92. Diagram to illustrate the sweep mode of operation to obtain a scalar tracing.

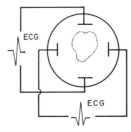

Fig. 1-93. Diagram to illustrate the vector mode of operation to obtain a loop.

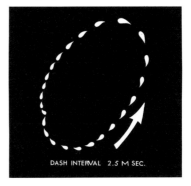

Fig. 1-94. Diagram showing teardrop-shaped dashes provided at 2.5 msec. interval.

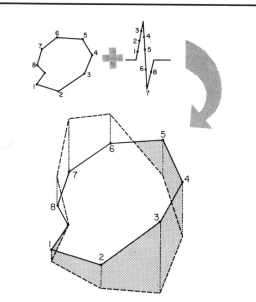

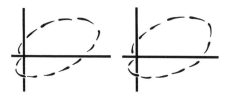

Fig. 1-95. Diagram showing the horizontal plane loop modulated by the Y lead amplitude at 8 points to get the illusion of seeing a loop as if it were traced in a 3-dimensional space.

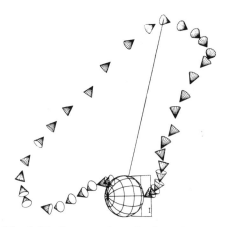

Fig. 1-96. Spatial image of the vector loop obtained from the 2 stereoscopic pictures to be viewed from a distance of approximately one foot with crossed lines of vision (convergence) so that the left eye is focused on the right-hand picture and vice versa.

Displaying Three-Dimensional Loops

The illusion of seeing a vector loop as if it were traced in a three-dimensional space is achieved by employing a number of different techniques. The simplest method is to modulate the horizontal vector loop by a vertical coordinate Y in a fully synchronized manner. When the amplitude of the Y lead is positive, the loop is modulated downward, and when the amplitude of the Y lead is negative, the loop is modulated upward (Fig. 1-95).

Another method is based on a stereo effect. In this method two related views are produced: one for the left eye in one projection plane, and the other for the right eye in another projection plane. These planes intersect at an angle that is normally set at 7.5°. This angle is approximately the eye-separation angle subtended at a point in space 500 mm from the eyes, when the interpupillary distance is 67 mm. Stereo viewing is achieved by permitting the left eye to see only the left-eye view and similarly for the right-eye view (Fig. 1-96).

Still another method is based on the drawing of solid figures at different angles, which depict the direction and orientation of a three-dimensional vectorcardiogram. This is accomplished by generating every 2 msec. a cone that has an advancing base and a trailing apex. Its outer surface is striped and the inner is white. The base of the cone is centered on the point generator of the loop, and when this point is moving toward the observer he sees mainly the base (i.e., the white inner surface) but when this point is moving outward from the observer, he sees mainly the apex and the striped outer surface. For all intermediate directions, a proper perspective of the cone is calculated (Fig. 1-97). The second and third methods require many operations (rotation of axes, translating the point of origin, etc.) that must be carried out by a computer, which subsequently drives a cathode-ray tube (oscilloscope).

Fig. 1-97. Construction of a three dimensional vector loop by generating cones at different angles (courtesy of Dr. L. Brinberg).

RESOLVER

Transformation of Coordinates

An instrument that performs the rotation of orthogonal axes, or more properly, the transformation of coordinates X, Y, Z into another orthogonal set X′, Y′, Z′, is called a resolver. This transformation is carried out according to mathematical formulas stated below. Rotation around the vertical axis Y by angle ϕ results in new coordinates (Fig. 1-98):

$$X' = X \cos \phi - Z \sin \phi$$
$$Z' = X \sin \phi + Z \cos \phi \qquad (1)$$

Rotation around X′ axis by angle θ results in new coordinates (Fig. 1-99):

$$Y' = Y \cos \theta - Z' \sin \theta$$
$$Z'' = Y \sin \theta + Z' \cos \theta \qquad (2)$$

The above mentioned mathematical formulas are more readily understood with the help of Figure 1-100.

Thus, by changing the azimuth angle ϕ and the elevation angle θ, one can rotate the reference frame XYZ to the desired new position X′Y′Z″. This rotation is accomplished by means of sine-cosine potentiometers as indicated in Figure 1-101.

For illustrative purpose, let us consider a point P, which in the original reference system XYZ is determined by coordinates X = 4, Y = 3, Z = 2. After this system has been rotated around Y axis by angle $\phi = 30°$, the same point P in space is then expressed by new coordinates:

$$X' = 4 \cos 30° - 2 \sin 30° = 2.5$$
$$Z' = 4 \sin 30° + 2 \cos 30° = 3.7$$

By further rotation of the coordinate system around a new axis X′ by angle $\theta = 60°$, the point P accepts the following coordinates:

$$Y' = 3 \cos 60° - 2 \sin 60° = -0.2$$
$$Z'' = 3 \sin 60° + 2 \cos 60° = 3.6.$$

Consequently, the coordinates of point P in the system, resulting from double rotation, are as follows: Z = 2.5, Y = −0.2, Z − 3.6.

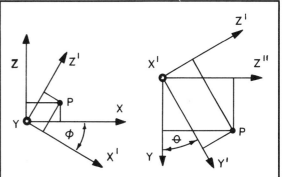

Fig. 1-98. (left) Rotation of X and Z coordinates around the vertical axis Y by an angle ϕ.

Fig. 1-99. (right) Rotation of Y and Z coordinates around horizontal axis X^1 by an angle Θ.

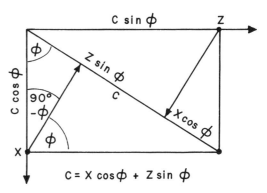

Fig. 1-100. Diagram illustrating the mathematical formula for rotation of a coordinate.

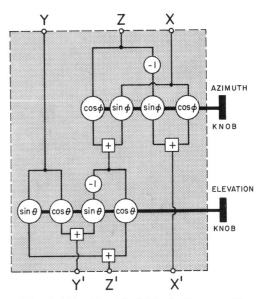

Fig. 1-101. Simplified block diagram illustrating basic elements employed by the instrument performing transformation of coordinates.

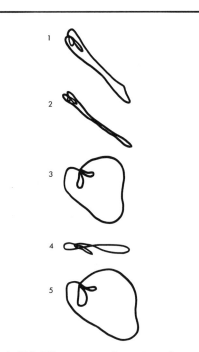

Fig. 1-102. The course of rotation of a vector-cardiographic loop: (1) the frontal plane VCG loop; (2) the edgewise projection in the frontal plane; (3) the horizontal plane VCG loop; (4) the edgewise projection in the horizontal plane; (5) the broadside projection in the horizontal plane.

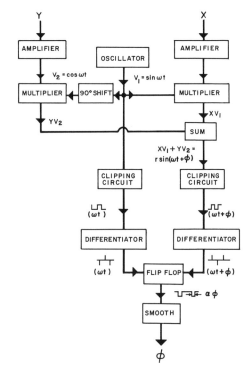

Fig. 1-103. Simplified block diagram of the electrical circuit which calculates an angle ϕ.

Rotation of Vectorcardiographic Loops

Several different procedures can be used to rotate QRS loops. It is convenient to start, for example, with the frontal loop, which by means of the azimuth angle dial can be rotated to an almost straight line ("edgewise" projection). The process is expressed by the equation (1) on page 43.

Symbol ϕ stands for an azimuth and X′, Z′ are the transformed coordinates. The rotation is made about axis Y, and, therefore, the coordinates X and Z are changed. The angle ϕ, or azimuth, is read off on the resolver.

From the "edgewise" projection of the frontal plane, one can rotate the azimuth angle dial by 90° to get the most open ("broadside") projection of the loop. The broadside projection of the frontal loop can be rotated about the X axis by twisting the knob for elevation angle. This operation is described by the equation (2) on the preceding page.

Symbol θ stands for elevation and Y′ and Z″ are the transformed coordinates. The rotation is made until an "edgewise" projection of the horizontal loop is obtained. From this position one gets a broadside projection of the QRS loop in a horizontal plane by rotating the elevation angle dial by 90° (Fig. 1-102).

The "viewpoint" for this projection can be read directly from the dials in terms of azimuth and elevation angles. These angles are identical with the spatial orientation of the polar vector. The ratio between the major and minor axes of the "edgewise" projection indicates the degree of planarity of the QRS loop. The ratio between the major and minor axes in the broadside projection characterizes the configuration of the QRS loop.

The coordinate rotation concept developed from the observation that the VCG loop in three-dimensional space is essentially planar for the QRS complex in normal subjects; and it represents another approach to the problem of eliminating apparent differences in vectorcardiograms of normal subjects, resulting from the orientation of the heart.

POLARCARDIOGRAPH

Principle of Operation

Recording polar coordinates of the heart vector against time yields graphs, which are called polarcardiograms. The instrument which makes possible such recording is called the polarcardiograph. The polarcardiograph computes polar coordinates of the heart vector from X, Y, and Z signals (or coordinates), and this transformation is accomplished according to certain mathematical formulas (see page 22) that may be simulated by electrical methods. One of these methods is described here. It employs an oscillator of frequency ω radians per second which generates a signal V_1, and through 90° shifts, a signal V_2. These signals are multiplied by signals X and Y respectively, and added according to the equation:

$$XV_1 + YV_2 = m \cos \phi \sin \omega t + m \sin \phi \cos \omega t$$
$$= m \sin (\omega t + \phi)$$

where m is the magnitude and ϕ the direction (azimuth) of the frontal plane heart vector.

To obtain ϕ, the effect of the varying m must be removed. This removal is achieved by amplifying and clipping so that the sine wave is converted into a square wave of identical phase, which is then differentiated to produce a train of alternating positive and negative pulses. A similar process of amplifying, clipping, and differentiating is carried out upon the oscillator output V_2, to give a second train of pulses, the phase of which differs from that of the first set by ϕ. The two trains are used to switch a bistable circuit, or flip-flop, which gives a train of rectangular pulses, the duration of which is proportional to ϕ. The larger the phase angle, ϕ, or time difference between the two trains driving the flip-flop, the greater the area of each of the rectangular pulses at the flip-flop output. Smoothing this output yields a voltage proportional to ϕ (Fig. 1-103).

The spatial magnitude M, and the polar angle (elevation) are obtained by adding another circuit (similar to that described above), which generates signal V_3 by filtering and shifting the square wave of phase $(\omega t + \phi)$, available from the previous operation. Signal V_3 is then multiplied by the signal Z and combined with XV_1 and XV_2 according to the equation

$$XV_1 + YV_2 + ZV_3 = m \sin(\omega t + \phi) + z \cos(\omega t + \phi)$$
$$= M[\sin \theta \sin(\omega t + \phi) + \cos \theta \cos(\omega t + \phi)]$$
$$= M \cos(\omega t + \phi - \theta)$$

where M is the magnitude of the heart spatial vector, and θ corresponds to its elevation. The spatial magnitude is extracted from the signal $M \cos(\omega t + \phi - \theta)$ by linear detection. The amplifying and clipping of the same signal eliminates the effect of the variation of M and yields a square wave of phase $(\omega t + \phi - \theta)$. Adding this to the square wave of phase $(\omega t + \phi)$, previously mentioned, yields a train of positive and negative rectangular pulses with areas proportional to θ, so that θ is then obtained by rectifying and smoothing the pulses, as was done for ϕ.

Time Plots of Polar Coordinates

Polar coordinates of the heart vector can be recorded both in space and also in a given plane. In space, the heart vector has the following polar coordinates: magnitude (M), azimuth (ϕ) and elevation (θ). In each plane there are only two polar coordinates: magnitude (m) and an angle of direction. This angle is often referred to as an azimuth, so one may speak of azimuth in the frontal, horizontal and sagittal planes respectively. According to another terminology, the angle of the heart vector in the frontal, horizontal and sagittal planes is called α, β, and γ respectively.

The time plot of the spatial magnitude of the heart vector resembles the R wave of an electrocardiographic tracing, because it does not have any negative deflections. Azimuth is plotted on the scale that reads zero in the center and ∓ 180 at the extremities. Elevation is plotted on the scale that reads zero in the center and ∓ 90 at the extremities (Fig. 1-104). These scales are described in more detail on page 51.

The transformation of the coordinates of the heart vector from rectangular to polar is merely a mathematical ma-

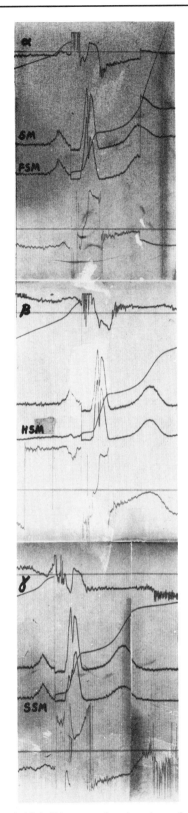

Fig. 1-104. Diagram showing time plots of polar coordinates. SM—spatial magnitude.

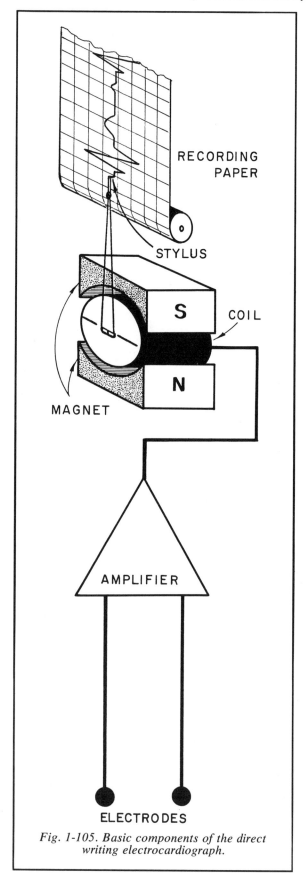

RECORDING
PAPER

STYLUS

S

COIL

N

MAGNET

AMPLIFIER

ELECTRODES

Fig. 1-105. Basic components of the direct writing electrocardiograph.

nipulation, and from the theoretical point of view it should not add any new information. However, recording polar coordinates has the advantage of preserving a time sequencing of electrical events in a heart cycle, which is not so evident in vector loops. This technique also gives a better picture of events close to the point J, which is often blurred because of a telescoping of the time dimension. The clinical value of angular information about the position of the heart vector during the heart cycle has not yet been assessed, because lack of suitable instrumentation has prevented the accumulation of sufficient data.

ELECTROCARDIOGRAPH

Components

An electrocardiograph machine consists of four main components: the primary circuit from the subject, an amplifier, a galvanometer, and the write-out mechanism effected through the galvanometer (Fig. 1-105). The electrical currents picked up by means of electrodes from the body surface pass to an amplifier, and after being amplified they activate a galvanometer. The resulting magnetic field oscillates a recording lever carrying either a thermostylus, which forms a trace by heating a specially prepared paper surface, or a pen which inscribes a trace on paper. When the positive potential is being recorded, the stylus (or pen) moves upward, thus inscribing a positive deflection; when the negative potential is being recorded, the stylus (or pen) moves downward, thus inscribing a negative deflection.

The above described instruments are called direct-writing electrocardiographs. However, still in use are so-called optical electrocardiographs.

In these instruments there is a coil of wire suspended in the magnetic field; a mirror is attached to the middle of the coil so that it oscillates when the coil oscillates. If a beam of light is played on the mirror as the coil oscillates, the reflected beam of light moves accordingly. This reflected beam of light can then be recorded on moving photographic paper (Fig. 1-106).

While in direct-writing electrocardiographs the records are available immediately, the optical type requires a development process which results in some delay. If, however, an ultraviolet-sensitive paper is used for recording, a readable chart is available within a few seconds of exposure to daylight. Instruments with optical registration have one big advantage of having a frequency response to 400 cps. The direct-writing electrocardiographs are capable of responding linearly only up to 100 cps.

The quality of an electrocardiograph can be tested by checking its frequency fidelity characterized by the response time and fade-out time. The response time (i.e., the time elapsing up to full response to constant calibration potential) is a measure of the correct registration of higher frequencies and must not exceed 0.01 sec. with an applied calibration potential of 1 mv. The fade-out time (i.e., the time required for a deflection to fall to the fraction $\frac{1}{2.72}$ of its initial amplitude) is an indication of the correct registration of lower frequencies and should not exceed 1.5 sec.

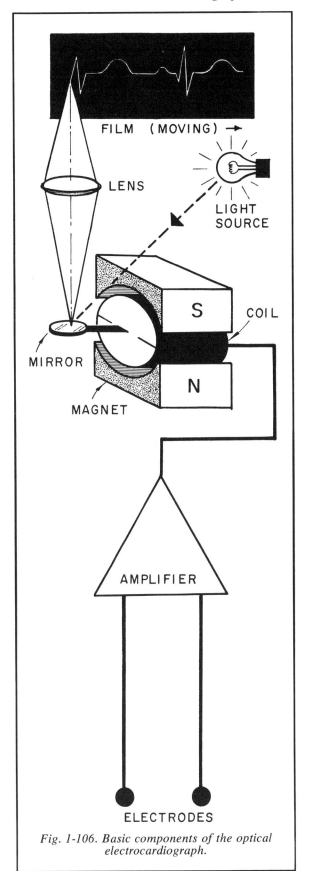

Fig. 1-106. Basic components of the optical electrocardiograph.

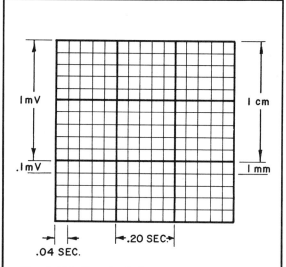

Fig. 1-107. *Standard electrocardiographic grid.*

STANDARDIZATION
DEFLECTION

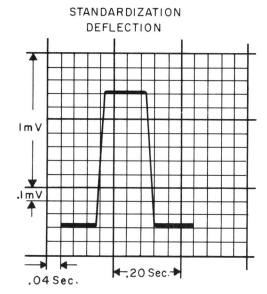

Fig. 1-108. *The standardization deflection of 10 mm (or 1 millivolt).*

Strip Chart Record

The electrocardiograph is used to record the heart electrical activity, as it is reflected in the conventional 12 lead system. This recording is accomplished on 50 mm heat sensitive paper which turns black when it is exposed to the stylus, whose tip is heated by electrical current. Consequently, this results in a black line at points on the paper that the stylus touches.

A standard grid superimposed on the recording paper consists of horizontal and vertical lines 1 mm apart; every fifth line is bolder than others, in order to facilitate the calculation of time and voltage measurements (Fig. 1-107). The distance between two thin horizontal lines corresponds to 0.1 mv; the distance between two thin vertical lines corresponds to 0.04 sec. The paper speed is 25 mm per second but in most ECG machines it can be adjusted to 50, 70 or 100 mm per second.

Before recording the ECG, the electrocardiograph machine is standardized by the use of a self-contained 1 mv impulse, to inscribe a deflection of 10 mm (Fig. 1-108). If the amplitude of the ECG tracing is too high, the standardization deflection may be halved. The standardization enables the amplitudes of the ECG tracing to be read off in millivolts.

When the heart is at rest, the electrocardiogram displays a straight horizontal line, a so-called isoelectric line or base line. This base line represents a constant value of the direct current, produced by the recording device. Alternating current developed with myocardial activity is superimposed upon this base line and is recorded as upward (positive), or downward (negative) deflections. The base line may be shifted whenever there is movement of electrodes or a sudden change in skin resistance. In such a case, the electrocardiographic signal is superimposed upon the base line variations.

Methods of Analyzing Electrical Activity of the Heart

REFERENCE FRAME FOR VECTORCARDIOGRAPHY

Rectangular Coordinates

By appropriate placement of electrodes and by coupling them with resistors, one can obtain three mutually perpendicular (orthogonal) leads, lead X (horizontal), lead Y (vertical), and lead Z (sagittal), which may be regarded as rectangular (or Cartesian) coordinates. A common zero point of these coordinates is superimposed upon the point of origin of the heart vector representing the cardiac dipole.

These orthogonal lead axes or Cartesian axes are oriented in the following way: X is positive leftward, Y is positive downward, and Z is positive backward (Fig. 1-109). This orientation of the electrocardiographic coordinates axes differs from that used in analytical geometry, where positive axes have an anterior, leftward and superior direction. The semi-axes can be used to define 8 octants in the following way:

X	Y	Z		octant	
+	−	−	anterior,	left,	superior
+	+	−	anterior,	left,	inferior
−	−	−	anterior,	right,	superior
−	+	−	anterior,	right,	inferior
+	−	+	posterior	left,	superior
+	+	+	posterior,	left,	inferior
−	−	+	posterior,	right,	superior
−	+	+	posterior,	right,	inferior

A rectangular coordinate system forms three planes. The coordinate axes X and Y form the frontal plane, X and Z the horizontal plane, and Y and Z the sagittal plane (Fig. 1-110).

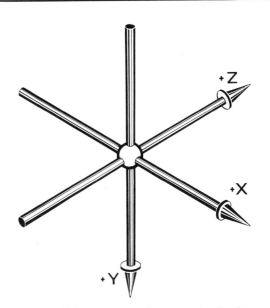

Fig. 1-109. A system of rectangular (orthogonal) coordinates representing the axes of leads used for recording the spatial heart vector.

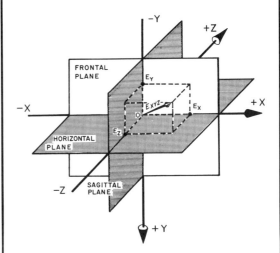

Fig. 1-110. Three planes as formed by the axes of X, Y, and Z leads.

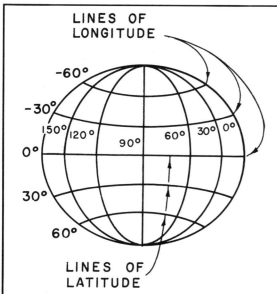

Fig. 1-111. *Diagram showing the geographic lines of latitude and longitude.*

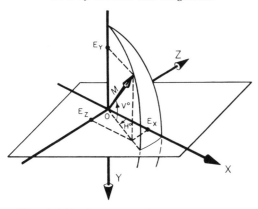

Fig. 1-112. *Diagram illustrating polar coordinates (M, H°, V°) of the heart vector in a 3-dimensional space.*

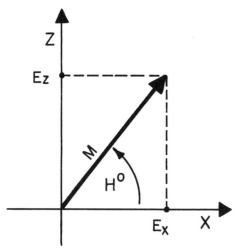

Fig. 1-113. *Diagram illustrating polar coordinates (M, H°) of the horizontal plane heart vector.*

Polar Coordinates

In addition to rectangular coordinates, one may use polar (or spherical) coordinates to define a location of the heart spatial vector. These coordinates are analogous to geographical lines of latitude and longitude and to the altitude, with respect to the center of the globe or to sea level (Fig. 1-111). However, in vectorcardiography the terms azimuth and elevation are used rather than longitude and latitude respectively. Also, instead of altitude, the term magnitude is employed in vectorcardiography. A position of the heart spatial vector can then be defined in terms of its magnitude, azimuth and elevation (Fig. 1-112). The magnitude of the heart spatial vector records the distance from the origin of the coordinate system to the tip of the vector. The azimuth angle is measured from the positive half of the X axis on the horizontal plane and the elevation angle is measured from the Z axis on the sagittal plane. The angular scale for these measurements is described below. The relationship between rectangular and polar coordinates is described on page 22.

It can easily be seen from Figure 1-113 that to define a position of the heart vector in a plane, only two polar coordinates are necessary, namely the magnitude and azimuth. Here, the azimuth angle is measured from a transverse axis, be it the X axis in the frontal or horizontal plane, or the Z axis in the sagittal plane. In order to conform to the nomenclature used by Einthoven, the pioneer of electrocardiography, the azimuth angle in the frontal plane is also called the angle α. Consequently, the azimuth angles in the horizontal and sagittal planes are also called the angle β and the angle γ respectively.

Angular Scale

For the purpose of indicating the direction of the cardiac vector in a plane, an angular scale is used. The angles in a plane are measured on a 0° to 360° scale or on a 0° to ±180° scale. The use of the latter system is recommended by the Committee on Standardization in Electrocardiography of the American Heart Association. It is also recommended that the angles be designated as follows: F° in the frontal plane, S° in the left sagittal plane, H° in the horizontal plane.

In the frontal plane 0° is set at the left extremity of the X axis and angles inscribed clockwise are positive from 0° to ±180° and those inscribed counterclockwise are negative from 0° to −180° (Fig. 1-114).

In the left sagittal plane (i.e., the plane viewed from the subject's left shoulder) a 0° is set at the posterior extremity of the Z axis and angles inscribed clockwise are positive from 0° to +180° and those inscribed counterclockwise are negative from 0° to −180° (Fig. 1-115). There is, as yet, a lack of uniform recording of the sagittal plane because many workers have been using the right sagittal plane. In the right sagittal (i.e., the plane viewed from the subject's right shoulder) a 0° is set at the anterior extremity of the Z axis and angles inscribed clockwise are positive from 0° to +180° and those inscribed counterclockwise are negative from 0° to −180° (Fig. 1-116).

In the horizontal plane a 0° is set at the left extremity of the X axis and angles inscribed clockwise are negative from 0° to −180°; and those inscribed counterclockwise are positive from 0° to +180° (Fig. 1-117).

To indicate the direction of the spatial heart vector, two angles are required, namely azimuth (H°) and elevation (V°). The azimuth is measured on the angular scale identical with that for the horizontal plane. The elevation is measured from the horizontal plane to the line connecting the origin and terminus of the spatial heart vector. Since this line can be projected on the sagittal plane, the angular scale in this plane is used for determining the elevation.

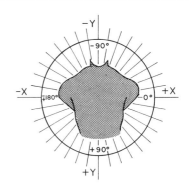

Fig. 1-114. Angular scale in the frontal plane.

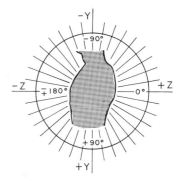

Fig. 1-115. Angular scale in the left sagittal plane.

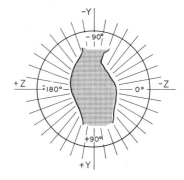

Fig. 1-116. Angular scale in the right sagittal plane.

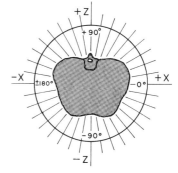

Fig. 1-117. Angular scale in the horizontal plane.

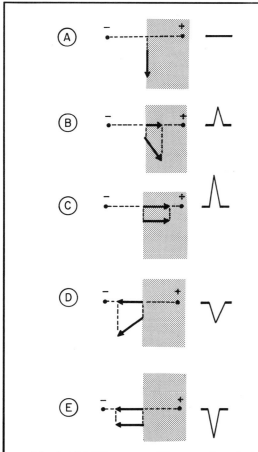

Fig. 1-118. Diagram to illustrate the relationship between the polarity and amplitude of the electrocardiographic deflection and the orientation and magnitude of the heart vector. The broken line represents the axis of the lead and the shadowed area the positive half of the axis. (A) Heart vector perpendicular to the lead axis; (B) heart vector projects on the positive side of the lead axis; (C) heart vector is parallel with the positive side of the lead axis; (D) heart vector projects on the negative side of the lead axis; (E) heart vector is parallel with the negative side of the lead axis.

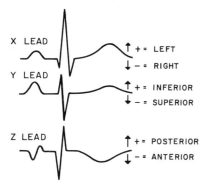

Fig. 1-119. Deflection in leads X, Y, and Z and their relation to the direction of the spatial heart vector.

ANALYSIS OF X, Y, AND Z COMPONENTS

Amplitude and Polarity of Deflections

Electrocardiographic deflections recorded in a given lead reflect the magnitude and direction of the particular heart spatial vector as it is projected on this lead axis. A simple way to look at this record is to consider the projection of the heart vector as its "shadow" on the lead axis, when there is a light source perpendicular to the axis of the lead. Consequently, the electrocardiographic deflection measures the size of the "shadow."

Amplitude of the electrocardiographic deflection is thus determined by the magnitude of the heart spatial vector, as well as by the angle that is extended between this vector and a given lead axis. If the heart spatial vector is perpendicular to a given lead axis, no deflection is recorded in this lead. If the heart spatial vector is parallel to a given lead axis, the largest deflection is recorded in this lead. Intermediate positions of the heart vector, in relation to the lead axis, result in deflections whose amplitude falls in the range between these two extremes.

Polarity of the electrocardiographic deflection depends on how the particular heart vector projects on the lead axis. If the particular heart vector projects onto the negative side of the lead axis, a negative deflection is recorded in this lead. Figure 1-118 shows the heart vector with four different directions relative to the lead axis, and the deflection which the lead records for each direction.

Since the ECG deflections represent the projection of the heart vector on a given lead axis, the direction and magnitude of the cardiac spatial vector are read from the ECG deflections. For example, an upward deflection in the lead X indicates that the cardiac vector is pointing to the left, a downward deflection in this lead indicates that the cardiac vector is pointing to the right (Fig. 1-119).

Terminology of Deflections

As the direction and magnitude of the cardiac spatial vector change from moment to moment in the course of a single cardiac cycle, the changes account for the characteristic pattern of potential variations recorded in leads X, Y, and Z (or any other leads). This pattern represents a curve consisting of 3 distinctive deflections and is called an electrocardiogram (Fig. 1-120).

The first deflection, designated as the P wave, is due to depolarization of the atria and marks the onset of atrial depolarization. The P wave may assume many shapes as shown in Figure 1-123. When the P wave is upright it is said to be positive; when downward, it is negative. When the P wave displays 2 peaks of different polarity it is said to be diphasic; the order of those peaks decides of the type of the diphasic P wave. Under certain circumstances the P wave may be flat, notched or absent (i.e., isoelectric).

Repolarization of the atria, designated as the T_a or T_p wave, is usually partially buried in the QRS deflection and may or may not be seen. If visible, it represents a small deflection whose polarity is opposite from that of the P wave (Fig. 1-121).

The second deflection, called the QRS complex, is due to depolarization of the ventricles and marks the onset of ventricular contraction. The QRS complex consists of one or more deflections, which are defined here.

1. Any positive deflection is called an R wave; if there is more than one, the second is labeled R′ (R prime).

2. A negative deflection is termed a Q wave if it precedes an R wave, and an S wave if it follows an R wave. A negative deflection that follows an R′ is called an S′ (S prime). The QRS complex in the form of a single negative deflection is referred to as a QS wave (or complex).

This terminology is illustrated in Fig. 1-122. Small deflections, generally under .5 mm, are usually written in lower-case letters, q, r, and s.

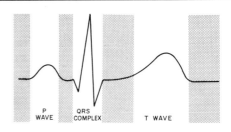

Fig. 1-120. Diagram showing significant components, namely the P wave, the QRS complex and the T wave of the normal scalar tracing (electrocardiogram).

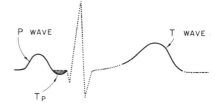

Fig. 1-121. Diagram showing the P wave, T_p wave, and T wave.

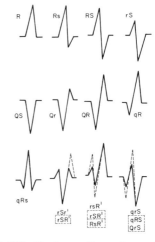

Fig. 1-122. Basic configurations of the QRS complex. The dashed line indicates the possibility of a bigger deflection occurring which will lead to another designation (written inside the dashed rectangle).

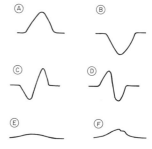

Fig. 1-123. Diagram showing various configurations of the P wave and T wave. (A) Positive; (B) Negative; (C) Diphasic (−+ type); (D) Diphasic (+− type); (E) Flat; (F) Notched.

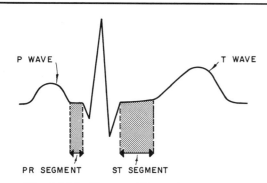

Fig. 1-124. Diagram illustrating various segments of the normal scalar tracing (electrocardiogram).

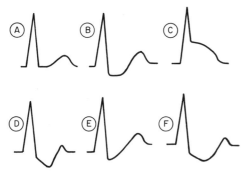

Fig. 1-125. Diagram showing various ST segment configurations. (A) Isoelectric; (B) depressed; (C) elevated; (D) downward sloping; (E) upward sloping; (F) "cupped".

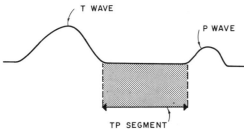

Fig. 1-126. The TP segment between the end of the T wave and the beginning of the P wave in the adjacent cycle.

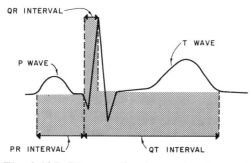

Fig. 1-127. Diagram showing various intervals of the normal scalar tracing (electrocardiogram).

The third deflection, called the T wave, is due to repolarization of the ventricles and coincides with the resting phase of the ventricles. The T wave may assume many shapes which have been designated in the same way as for the P wave (Fig. 1-123). Thus one speaks of the positive T wave when it is upright or the negative T wave when it is downward, etc.

Segments and Intervals

Isoelectric portions of the electrocardiogram (i.e., periods when no potential is recorded), are called segments and are designated by the letters of the preceding and following deflections. That part of the tracing which lies between the end of the P wave and the onset of the QRS complex is called a PR or PQ segment (Fig. 1-124). It is normally isoelectric or slightly negative. A considerable depression of this segment is called an atrial repolarization wave (T_a).

The ST segment lies between the end of the QRS complex and the beginning of the T wave; and it corresponds to the period of complete ventricular depolarization (Fig. 1-124). It is usually isoelectric but in lead Z and the precordial leads an elevation of 2 mm or a depression of 0.05 mm is normal. In tachycardia the ST segment may start slightly low but then climbs steadily, resulting in an upward sloping configuration. On the other hand, when the S wave is absent the ST segment often starts slightly high from the descending limb of the R wave, resulting in a downward sloping configuration. Different configurations of the ST segment are shown in Figure 1-125. The point where the QRS ends and ST segment begins is referred to as J (junction) point.

Between the end of the T wave and the beginning of the P wave in the adjacent cycle there is the TP segment. This segment is almost always isoelectric and is usually taken as a reference for a base line (Fig. 1-126).

A segment together with the preceding and/or following wave is called an interval. The PQ (or PR) interval is measured from the beginning of the P wave to the beginning of the QRS complex (Fig. 1-127). This interval represents the time required for depolarization of the atria, as well as that involved in the physiological delay in the conduction of the impulse by the atrioventricular node; it is partly dependent on the heart rate (a higher heart rate is accompanied by a shorter PQ interval).

The QR interval, called also an intrinsicoid deflection onset, is measured from the beginning of the QRS complex to the peak of R (or R′) where the signal starts to fall (Fig. 1-127). This period is the time consumed by the spread of the depolarization wave from the endocardium to the epicardial surface.

The QT interval denotes the time elapsing during depolarization and repolarization of the ventricles and is measured from the start of the QRS complex to the end of the T wave (Fig. 1-127).

ANALYSIS OF VECTOR LOOPS

Construction of a Vector Loop

A vector loop is constructed by plotting at the right angle any two orthogonal leads recorded simultaneously. For example, the frontal plane vector loop is constructed from the X and Y leads, as shown in Figure 1-128. The successive instantaneous potentials in the X and Y leads at intervals of 0.01 second are plotted on the axes of the leads and from these points perpendiculars are dropped. The intersection of each pair of perpendicular lines corresponds to the tip of an instantaneous horizontal plane vector drawn from the center of the reference frame. When the calculated positions of successive, instantaneous vectors are connected by a line beginning and terminating at the center of the planar reference frame, a frontal vector loop is obtained. Obviously, the greater the number of successive instantaneous potentials in the X and Y leads, the more accurate is the construction of the frontal plane vector loop. In a similar way, one constructs the horizontal plane loop from the X and Z leads, and the sagittal plane loop from the Y and Z leads.

Direct registration of vector loops is carried out by means of a cathode-ray oscilloscope where the loop appears on the fluorescent screen and are photographed directly. This is accomplished by connecting one orthogonal lead to the horizontal plates and another orthogonal lead to the vertical plates of the oscilloscope (for details see page 41).

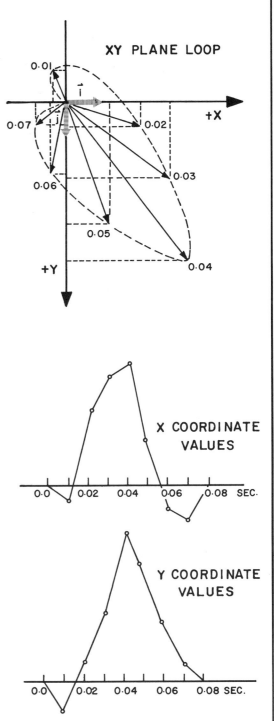

Fig. 1-128. Diagram to illustrate the construction of a vector loop in the frontal (XY) plane using X and Y coordinate values at t = 0.00, 0.01, 0.02, 0.03, 0.04, 0.05, 0.06, 0.07, and 0.08 sec. Each instantaneous vector in the XY plane is obtained by vectorial summation of corresponding vectors directed along X and Y axis.

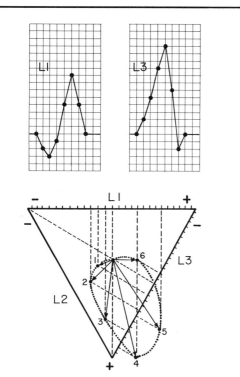

Fig. 1-129. Diagram illustrating the construction of the frontal plane vector loop from 2 bipolar limb leads (L1 and L3).

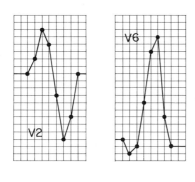

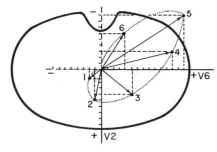

Fig. 1-130. Diagram illustrating the construction of the horizontal plane vector loop from 2 precordial (V2 and V5) leads.

A vector loop also can be constructed from leads which are not orthogonal. For example, the frontal plane vector loop would be constructed from any two of the bipolar or unipolar limb leads (Fig. 1-129); and the horizontal plane vector loop from any two precordial leads (Fig. 1-130). The most serious objection for doing this is that these leads are recorded sequentially; thus, they lack phase information, which is provided by simultaneous recording. However, despite the inaccuracy of the method, the attempt to visualize the 12 lead system electrocardiograms in terms of vector loops is helpful in understanding and interpreting electrocardiographic patterns.

P Vector Loop

Detailed analysis of the P loop cannot be performed unless great magnification is available. In such cases, the P loop is described in terms of its shape, direction of inscription, and the magnitude and orientation of the maximum P vector (Fig. 1-131). This terminology is similar to that applied to the QRS loop and is discussed on page 57.

The P loop starts at the E point and ends at the 0 point, which is located superiorly, slightly posteriorly and rightward in respect to the E point. Since, at the E point the electron beam of the oscilloscope remains stationary for the time when no electrical activity exists (i.e., during the ST segment and TP interval), the photographed image of this point is usually much brighter than the loops and may defeat precise measuring of the P wave loop parameters.

The line segment from the E point to the 0 point represents the atrial repolarization (or T_a) vector; this vector is usually opposite to the direction of the mean or maximum P vector (Fig. 1-132).

QRS Vector Loop

The QRS loop may be analyzed in the following terms:

1. The direction and speed of inscription of the loop;
2. The configuration of the loop;
3. The magnitude and direction of instantaneous QRS vectors.

The direction of inscription of the QRS loop is indicated by a thicker, brighter portion of dashes making up the pattern and is described as either clockwise (CW), counterclockwise (CCW), or figure-of-eight (Fig. 1-133); the latter is further described by referring to the direction of inscription of initial portion.

The speed of inscription is judged from the distance between dashes, which usually is 2 msec. Normally, the QRS loop is inscribed with a more or less constant speed. Slowing of the QRS loop is indicated by the dashes being closely spaced (Fig. 1-134). However, a normal loop may appear to be slowly inscribed in the plane perpendicular to the heart vector, so that there should be slowing in at least two planes to be certain that slowed conduction actually exists.

The configuration of the QRS loop is usually expressed in purely descriptive terms, which refer either to the loop area or to the relation of the loop to the recording axes.

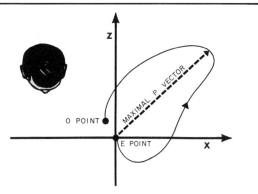

Fig. 1-131. Diagram illustrating main features of the P loop.

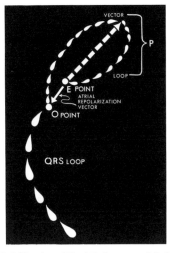

Fig. 1-132. Amplified P loop and initial portion of the QRS loop to demonstrate the atrial repolarization vector (T_a).

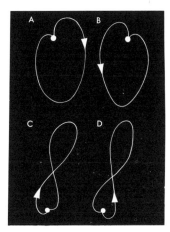

Fig. 1-133. Diagram to illustrate different directions of inscription of the QRS loop. (A) CW inscription; (B) CCW inscription; (C) figure-of-eight with the initial portion inscribed CW; (D) figure-of-eight with the initial portion inscribed CCW.

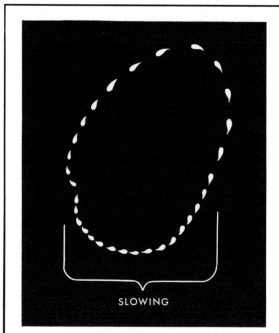

Fig. 1-134. Diagram to illustrate the slowing of the QRS loop.

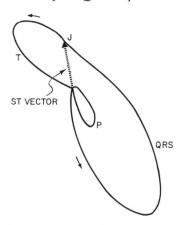

Fig. 1-135. Diagram illustrating the formation of an ST vector when the QRS loop does not "close" (i.e., does not return to the point E).

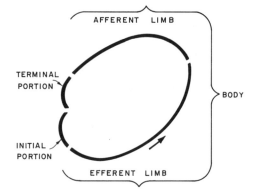

Fig. 1-136. Diagram showing the main divisions of the QRS loop.

The following terms are used for describing the QRS loop configuration: round, oval, elongated, figure-of-eight, pulled forward and to the left, pulled backward and to the right, etc. In addition, the QRS loop may be closed or open. Normally, repolarization begins a short period after depolarization ends, so that the QRS loop starts and ends at the same point, which is called 0 point. This point is slightly separated from the isoelectric point (E point) because of the atrial repolarization vector. If, however, repolarization of ventricles begins before their depolarization ends the QRS loop does not return to the point of origin, because the resting electrical state has failed to appear. The loop opens and the ST vector, between the origin and the terminus of the QRS loop (or the orifice of the T loop), is present (Fig. 1-135). Unless the magnitude of the ST vector is abnormally increased, this vector can be identified only when great amplification is used.

An important feature that is often described is the QRS loop contour. The QRS contour is usually smooth but the loop may be marked by one or more "scallops" or "bulges" (see page 116). These scallops usually reflect a sudden change of the heart vector propagation and are believed to be related to small areas of fibrosis.

Another way of describing the QRS loop configuration is to divide it into initial portion, body and terminal portion, and to describe the magnitude and orientation of each part. The initial portion, sometimes called the Q loop, is arbitrarily defined as the very first deflection of the QRS loop produced by vectors appearing during the first 10 to 20 msec. after the onset of ventricular depolarization. The body of the QRS loop, sometimes called the R loop, constitues the major portion of the QRS loop. It consists of two limbs, the efferent (or outgoing) limb and the afferent (or returning) limb, which are separated by the turning point of the loop. The terminal portion, sometimes called the S loop, is arbitrarily defined as the last portion of the QRS loop produced by vectors appearing during the last 15 msec. of ventricular depolarization (Fig. 1-136).

Dividing the QRS loop into initial portion, efferent limb, afferent limb, and terminal portion is mainly a matter of individual judgment, and therefore the division is not very accurate. More precise analysis of the QRS loop is achieved by measuring the magnitude and direction of QRS vectors. Vectors arising from the 0 point (origin) and ending at any point of the vector loop are labeled instantaneous QRS vectors (see page 26). These vectors are calculated at fixed intervals from the beginning of the QRS loop. Usually five initial vectors at 0.00, 0.01, 0.02, 0.03, and 0.04 sec. from the beginning of ventricular depolarization, and five terminal vectors at 0.04, 0.03, 0.02, 0.01, and 0.00 sec. before end of ventricular depolarization are analyzed. Due to the inter-individual variability in duration of ventricular depolarization, those vectors may overlap or lead to a gap in the middle part of the QRS loop. In order to overcome this difficulty, one may use time normalized instantaneous QRS vectors. In this case the ventricular depolarization, regardless of its duration, is represented by five or eight instantaneous vectors equally spaced (Fig. 1-137).

The most important among instantaneous vectors of the QRS loop is the maximum QRS vector, which is identical with the major axis of the QRS loop. It starts at the point of origin and ends at the most remote point of the loop. The magnitude of the maximum QRS vector is proportional to its length, and the direction of this vector is defined as the angle subtended by the vector and the horizontal axis (Fig. 1-138). The maximum QRS vector is a rough approximation of the mean QRS vector. The latter represents the average magnitude and direction of all instantaneous QRS vectors, and is calculated using planimeter. Better approximation of the mean QRS vector is obtained by calculating the half-area vector (i.e., the vector which divides the QRS loop into two equal half-areas). Such a calculation also requires the use of planimeter.

Extremely important for QRS loop analysis is the initial QRS vector, which is the resultant vector representing the average magnitude and direction of QRS vectors generated during the first 10 or 20 msec. of the ventricular depolarization. This vector is usually calculated by dividing the area of the initial portion of the QRS loop into two approximately equal areas (Fig. 1-139). The magnitude and direction of this vector can be readily ascertained if one knows the calibration and the angular scale.

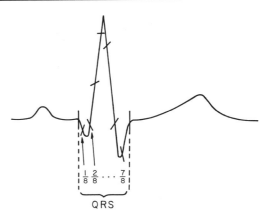

Fig. 1-137. Diagram to illustrate the division of the QRS loop into eight equal portions (instantaneous vectors).

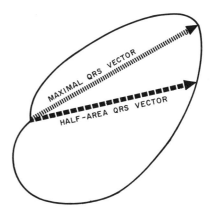

Fig. 1-138. Diagram to illustrate the concept of the maximal QRS vector and the half-area QRS vector.

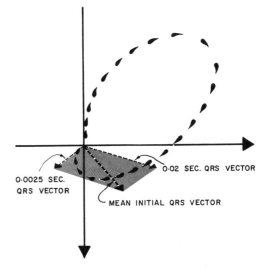

Fig. 1-139. Diagram illustrating the concept of the initial QRS vector. The first dot indicates the position of the 0.0025 sec. QRS vector; the eighth dot indicates the position of the 0.02 sec. QRS vector.

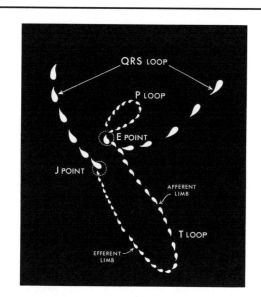

Fig. 1-140. Amplified T vector loop.

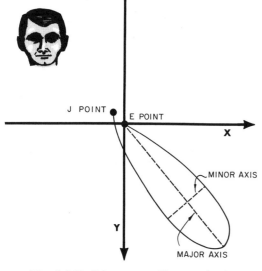

Fig. 1-141. Diagram to illustrate basic features of the T loop.

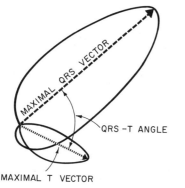

Fig. 1-142. Diagram to illustrate the concept of the planar QRS-T angle.

T Vector Loop

The T vector loop analysis involves determination of the direction and speed of inscription of the loop, the loop configuration, the direction and magnitude of the maximum T vector and the QRS-T angle. Determination of the direction and speed of inscription of the T loop is carried out in the same way as for the QRS loop. In some cases the direction of inscription of the T loop can be inferred from the fact that the initial portion of the T loop normally is inscribed at a slower rate than the terminal portion (Fig. 1-140). This initial slowing can be seen in many cases when the T loop is amplified x 2. Better visualization of the direction of inscription of the T loop can be obtained by increasing the duration between the drop-shaped dashes to 10 msec. instead of usual 2.5 msec.

The maximum T vector, or the major axis of the T loop, is measured from the E point to the most remote point of the T loop. Although the beginning of the T loop does not coincide with the E point, the latter has been chosen, since it is not affected by the ST vector. The line perpendicular to the major axis of the T loop at the point of maximal width is called the minor axis (Fig. 1-141). The shape of the T loop can be expressed by the major-axis to minor-axis ratio or the length-to-width ratio which normally is above 2.5.

The angle subtended by the maximum QRS vector and maximum T vector is called the QRS-T angle (Fig. 1-142). This angle is calculated by subtracting the angle of the maximum T vector from the angle of the maximum QRS vector. Theoretically, the QRS-T angle should be calculated between the mean QRS vector and the mean T vector, or at least between the half-area QRS vector and the half-area T vector. However, such calculations are time-consuming and not practical unless done by a computer.

ANALYSIS OF THE 12 LEAD SYSTEM ELECTROCARDIOGRAMS

Frontal Plane Leads

Analysis of the bipolar and unipolar limb leads involves measuring of the amplitude and duration of wave form components and this is carried out in a similar way as for X, Y, Z leads (see page 52). In addition, the so-called electrical axis of the heart is determined from these leads.

Since the bipolar and unipolar limb leads axes lie approximately in the frontal plane, it follows that these leads record the X and Y components of the cardiac spatial vector, or the projection of the cardiac spatial vector on the frontal plane. Thus, they can be used to calculate, in an approximate way, the magnitude and orientation of the mean QRS vector in the frontal plane (sometimes called the electrical axis of the heart). For this purpose, the bipolar limb lead axes are represented by the sides of an equilateral triangle, the so-called Einthoven's triangle. The apices of the triangle indicate the three lead points, the two arms and the left leg. The midpoint of each bipolar limb lead axis divides the axis into positive and negative halves. Perpendicular lines drawn through the centers of the lead axes of bipolar limb leads intersect at the center of the equilateral triangle, and from this point the dipole vector originates (Fig. 1-143).

For convenience, the equilateral triangle can be rearranged into a triaxial reference frame by translating the midpoints of the sides of the equilateral triangle to a common origin (Fig. 1-144). The axes of the triaxial reference frame intersect, making angles of 60°. Zero degrees is taken along the positive limb of lead 1. Positive angles to 180° are measured clockwise, and negative angles to −180° are measured counterclockwise.

The lead axis of unipolar limb lead is seen in the Einthoven triangle as a line which bisects the angle at an apex and passes through the center of the triangle, forming a perpendicular with the opposite side (Fig. 1-145). The axes of the unipolar leads form another triaxial reference system, which is rotated 30° from the bipolar reference system. By superimposing the center points of those two reference systems, a hexaxial reference system is obtained, which is divided into 30° segments (Fig. 1-146).

The mean QRS vector in the frontal plane is called an electrical axis of the heart and is denoted by the symbol $\overline{A}_{XY}^{QRS}$. Determination of the electrical axis is illustrated in Figure 1-147. The algebraic sums of the amplitudes of the positive and negative deflections at a given instant, in at least two of three bipolar leads, are plotted on the appropriate sides of the Einthoven's triangle (or triaxial reference frame), and perpendiculars are drawn at these points to the sides; the point of intersection then yields the mean vector or electrical axis.

A more exact method consists in measuring not amplitudes but the areas bounded by the QRS complex and the base line. The area of the QRS complex is calculated according to the formula: area = 1/2 width × height. The areas are positive above the base line and negative below the base line. For each QRS complex the positive and negative areas are added algebraically and the sums are plotted

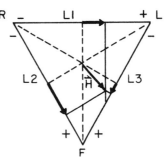

Fig. 1-143. The Einthoven equilateral triangle whose sides represent the axes (or lead vectors) of bipolar limb leads on which the frontal plane heart vector is projected.

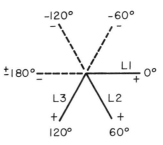

Fig. 1-144. Triaxial reference frame as formed by the axes of the bipolar limb leads shifted to intersect at the center of the triangle.

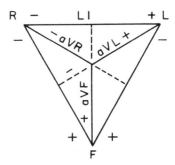

Fig. 1-145. The axes of the bipolar and unipolar limb leads as visualized in the Einthoven's equilateral triangle.

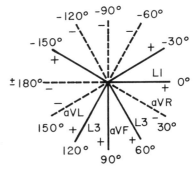

Fig. 1-146. Hexaxial reference frame as formed by the axes of the bipolar and unipolar limb leads in the Einthoven triangle.

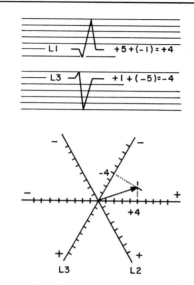

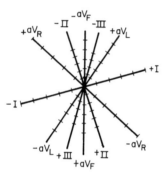

Fig. 1-147. Diagram to illustrate the calculation of the frontal plane mean QRS vector from leads L1 and L3.

Fig. 1-148. Diagram to illustrate the hexaxial reference frame based on the Burger triangle.

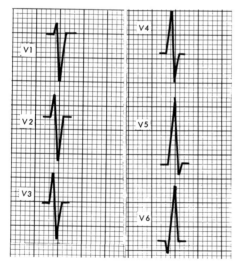

Fig. 1-149. Diagram showing the R/S progression observed in the precordial leads in normal subjects.

into the Einthoven triangle or the triaxial reference system, resulting in an electrical axis.

Since the advent of the concept of lead vectors it has been realized that more accurate results can be obtained by using a reference frame based on the Burger triangle (see page 37). The hexaxial system based on Burger's triangle is shown in Figure 1-148. The axes of this system have different scales to provide compensation for the unequal strength of the various leads. When the length of the scale unit on lead L1 is regarded as 1.0, the length of the scale unit on other leads can be expressed by the following proportionality factors: L2 = 0.6, L3 = 0.5, aVR = 1.1, aVL = 0.8, aVF = .06.

Horizontal Plane Leads

Precordial leads are analyzed in terms of the amplitude and duration of wave form components, in a similar way as was described for leads X, Y, and Z. In addition, the R/S progression across the precordium is inspected. Normally, it is a smooth progression from rS in V1 through RS in V2 and V3, and a qRS in V4 through V6 (Fig. 1-149).

When the precordial leads are studied, emphasis is placed upon the onset of the steepest downstroke of the R wave (intrinsicoid deflection). The onset of the intrinsicoid deflection corresponds to the QR interval (see page 54) and is believed to signal approximately the time of arrival of depolarization on the epicardial surface of that region of the ventricular wall which lies nearest to the precordial electrode. Delayed onset of the intrinsicoid deflection is characteristic of ventricular conduction defects and ventricular hypertrophy.

In the light of vectorial interpretation of the electrical activity of the heart, the axes of precordial leads can be considered as laying approximately in the horizontal plane. Thus, these leads record the X and Z components of the cardiac spatial vector or the projection of this vector on the horizontal plane. Hence, it appears that the potential difference in a precordial lead can be visualized as the projection of the spot describing the horizontal vector loop on that particular lead axis at a given instant. When the positions of these projected points on a given lead axis are plotted on an ordinate, while their time of occurrence is plotted on an abscissa, a classic electrocardiogram for that particular lead is obtained (Fig. 1-150). A similar relationship exists between limb leads and the frontal plane vector loop (Fig. 1-151).

In this way, from the vector loop, a rough prediction of the configuration of a given lead can be made; on the other hand, scalar electrocardiograms (in at least 2 leads) can be used to construct a rough approximation of the vectorcardiographic loop. However, this relationship is only approximate, since it is not possible to reconstruct accurately the phase relationship between 2 scalar leads recorded at different instances, and since assumptions are made regarding the axis of the standard and unipolar leads, which are only approximately correct.

Special research techniques confirm the presence of nondipolar content of precordial leads. However, this content is very small, relative to the error of placement of electrodes, and its diagnostic value is questionable.

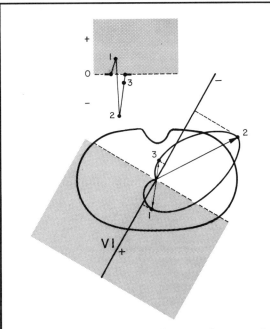

Fig. 1-150. Diagram to illustrate the manual derivation of the QRS complex in lead V1 from the horizontal plane QRS loop. For simplicity only 3 points on the loop were chosen to project on the axis of lead V1.

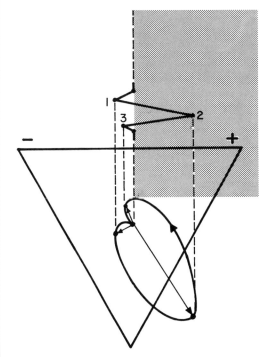

Fig. 1-151. Diagram to illustrate the manual derivation of the QRS complex in lead L1 from the frontal plane QRS loop using the equilateral triangle. For simplicity only 3 points on the loop were chosen to project on the axis of lead L1.

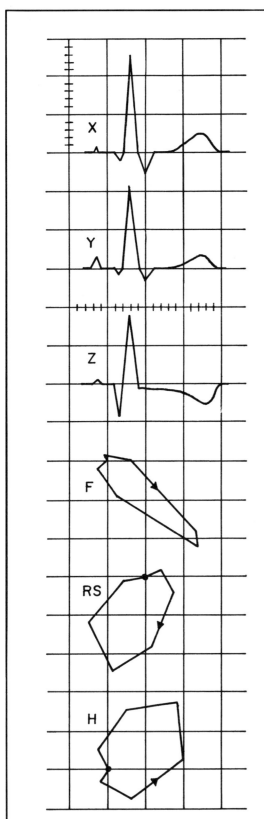

Fig. 1-152. Diagram showing the averaged X, Y, and Z leads and vector loops.

Normal Patterns of Electrical Activity of the Heart

NORMAL VECTORCARDIOGRAM

Appraisal of Normal VCG Data

The principles involved in determination of vectorcardiographic normal values have been described on page 146. So far no truly valid vectorcardiographic normal values are available. Standards for the normal vectorcardiogram, that have been proposed by several investigators, are far from being representative of the average clinically healthy population. For the most part this is due to the fact that the norms were derived from insufficient sampling of healthy subjects, and the normality was decided upon a single clinical examination at the time the VCG was taken. Because cardiovascular disease is widespread, one should expect that even a carefully examined group of healthy population will include some percentage of cardiac patients, thus introducing many false diagnoses of normality. It is obvious that establishing the representative sample of the normal population would be much more reliable if the definition of "health" was established in follow-up studies.

Another crucial factor to deal with is homogeneous samples. It is extremely desirable to stratify the total healthy human population according to constitutional variables (such as age, sex, race, weight, chest configuration, etc.), and calculate normal values for each group. The result is narrowing down of the wide range of distribution of vectorcardiographic items. Unfortunately, so far, the normal VCG values have been obtained from heterogeneous samples. The combination of heterogeneous groups, different in age, sex, race, and other constitutional and environmental variables, results in an increased range of distribution and a large overlap of patients with cardiac pathology.

Statistical Characteristics of the Normal VCG Data

The normal values of vectorcardiographic data presented here are based on those studies employing the Frank lead system in adults. This data, however, applies to a great extent to any other corrected orthogonal system, since the performance of such systems is relatively similar.

The normal values are generally presented as either the mean plus and minus the standard deviation (SD), or the mean and the lower and upper limit (Min → Max) of the 96 percent range. The latter specification is usually used in cases when the distribution is not symmetrical or normal (see page 147).

It is not enough to know the mean (or average) value, but also how much "variability" or "scatter" may exist about the mean so that it may still be considered "normal." In general, values lying within the mean ± two standard deviations might be considered "compatible with health," those falling between 2 and 3 standard deviations as "possibly indicative of disease," and those falling outside the 3 standard deviations as "probably indicative of disease." More sophisticated interpretation is discussed on page 148.

A representative vectorcardiogram in a healthy adult male is shown in Figure 1-152. In Tables 1-1—1-7 and Figures 1-153—1-158 are listed normal values of vectorcardiographic items obtained in 510 normal men using the orthogonal lead system of Frank. They were reported by Draper *et al.* in 1964 (Circulation *30*:853). Time intervals were measured in the manner discussed on page 159.

TABLE 1-1. NORMAL VALUES OF TIME INTERVALS (IN SECONDS)

ITEM	MEAN ± SD	MIN → MAX
P duration	0.102 ± 0.016	0.068 → 0.140
P-R interval	0.153 ± 0.023	0.112 → 0.204
P-R segment	0.051 ± 0.019	0.012 → 0.096
QRS duration	0.093 ± 0.009	0.076 → 0.112
Q-T interval	0.367 ± 0.448	0.312 → 0.448

TABLE 1-2. NORMAL VALUES OF THE P WAVE, QRS COMPLEX AND T WAVE IN LEAD X

ITEM		MEAN ± SD	MIN → MAX
P	amp. (mv)	0.06 ± 0.03	0.03 → 0.12
Q	amp. (mv)	0.10 ± 0.05	0.03 → 0.25
Q	dur. (sec.)	0.019 ± 0.004	0.012 → 0.028
R	amp. (mv)	1.17 ± 0.37	0.51 → 1.97
R	dur. (sec.)	0.051 ± 0.016	0.028 → 0.088
S	amp. (mv)	0.27 ± 0.15	0.06 → 0.68
S	dur. (sec.)	0.039 ± 0.008	0.024 → 0.056
J	amp.* (mv)	0.01 ± 0.03	−0.06 → 0.08
T	amp. (mv)	0.27 ± 0.13	0.06 → 0.56
Q/R	amp. ratio	0.08 ± 0.04	0.02 → 0.21
R	peak time (sec.)	0.037 ± 0.005	0.028 → 0.048

*Point J amplitude may be regarded as representative of the whole ST segment.

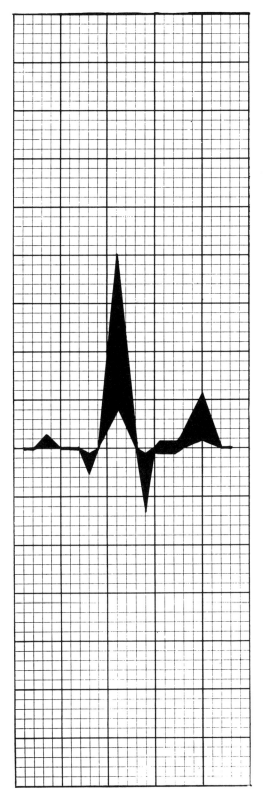

Fig. 1-153. Diagram to illustrate the 96 percent range of amplitude measurements (in mm) in lead X in 510 normal subjects.

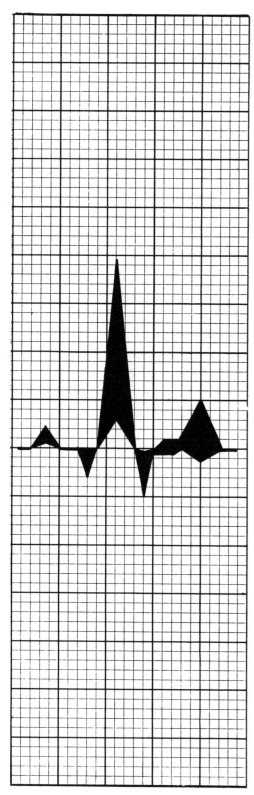

Fig. 1-154. Diagram to illustrate the 96 percent range of amplitude measurements (in mm) in lead Y in 510 normal subjects.

TABLE 1-3. NORMAL VALUES OF THE P WAVE, QRS COMPLEX AND T WAVE IN LEAD Y

ITEM		MEAN ± SD	MIN → MAX
P	amp. (mv)	0.11 ± 0.07	0.05 → 0.23
Q	amp. (mv)	0.10 ± 0.07	0.01 → 0.29
Q	dur. (sec.)	0.021 ± 0.005	0.008 → 0.032
R	amp. (mv)	1.03 ± 0.41	0.35 → 1.95
R	dur. (sec.)	0.061 ± 0.019	0.028 → 0.100
S	amp. (mv)	0.18 ± 0.12	0.03 → 0.49
S	dur. (sec.)	0.035 ± 0.010	0.020 → 0.056
J	amp.* (mv)	0.03 ± 0.04	−0.06 → 0.10
T	amp. (mv)	0.22 ± 0.13	−0.11 → 0.48
Q/R	amp. ratio	0.10 ± 0.05	0.01 → 0.22
R	peak time (sec.)	0.039 ± 0.005	0.028 → 0.052

*Point J amplitude may be regarded as representative of the whole ST segment.

TABLE 1-4. NORMAL VALUES OF THE P WAVE, QRS COMPLEX AND T WAVE IN LEAD Z

ITEM		MEAN ± SD	MIN → MAX
P	amp. (mv)	0.03 ± 0.05	−0.06 → 0.10
Q	amp. (mv)	0.41 ± 0.21	0.09 → 0.93
Q	dur. (sec.)	0.033 ± 0.007	0.020 → 0.048
R	amp. (mv)	0.93 ± 0.35	0.36 → 1.79
R	dur. (sec.)	0.059 ± 0.010	0.032 → 0.080
S	amp. (mv)		
S	dur. (sec.)		
J	amp.* (mv)	−0.07 ± 0.04	−0.17 → 0.00
T	amp. (mv)	−0.28 ± 0.13	−0.58 → 0.06
Q/R	amp. ratio	−0.49 ± 0.35	0.10 → 1.21
R	peak time (sec.)	0.049 ± 0.006	0.036 → 0.064

*Point J amplitude may be regarded as representative of the whole ST segment.

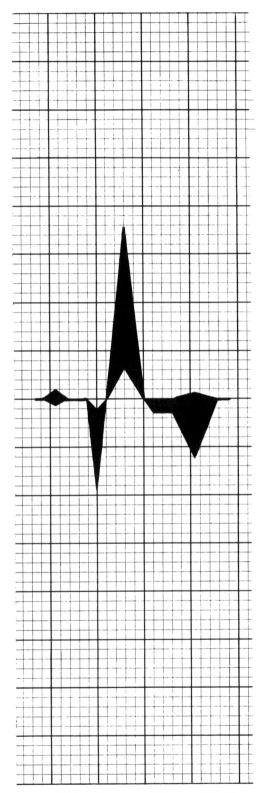

Fig. 1-155. Diagram to illustrate the 96 percent range of amplitude measurements (in mm) in lead Z in 510 normal subjects.

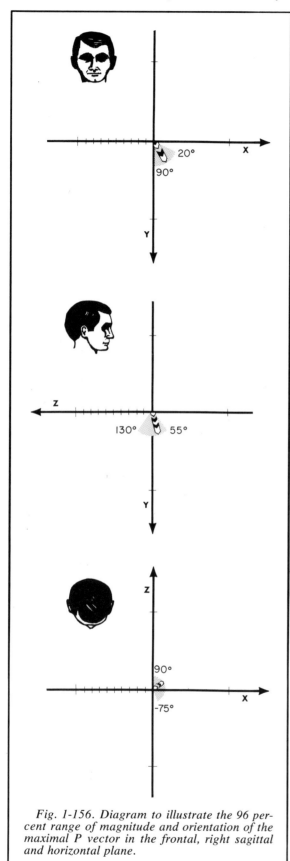

Fig. 1-156. Diagram to illustrate the 96 percent range of magnitude and orientation of the maximal P vector in the frontal, right sagittal and horizontal plane.

TABLE 1-5. NORMAL VALUES OF THE MAXIMAL P VECTOR MAGNITUDE (IN MILLIVOLTS) AND ORIENTATION (IN DEGREES)

		MEAN ± SD	MIN → MAX
3-Dimensional Space	amplitude	0.18 ± 0.06	0.09 → 0.32
	azimuth	−18° ± 38	−83° → 75°
	elevation	63° ± 17	20° → 86°
Frontal Plane	amplitude	0.18 ± 0.06	0.08 → 0.30
	azimuth	65° ± 18	20° → 90°
Right Sagittal Plane	amplitude	0.17 ± 0.06	0.06 → 0.30
	azimuth	85° ± 20	55° → 130°
Horizontal Plane	amplitude	0.09 ± 0.03	0.04 → 0.14
	azimuth	10° ± 40	−75° → 90°

TABLE 1-6. NORMAL VALUES OF THE MAXIMAL
QRS VECTOR MAGNITUDE (IN MILLIVOLTS)
AND ORIENTATION (IN DEGREES)

		MEAN ± SD	MIN → MAX
3-Dimensional Space	amplitude	1.73 ± 0.44	0.92 → 2.75
	azimuth	−29° ± 27	−97° → 23°
	elevation	35° ± 13	7° → 60°
Frontal Plane	amplitude	1.57 ± 0.42	0.81 → 2.53
	azimuth	40° ± 14	14° → 70°
Right Sagittal Plane	amplitude	1.32 ± 0.45	0.60 → 2.42
	azimuth	100° ± 30	50° → 165°
Horizontal Plane	amplitude	1.39 ± 0.36	0.74 → 2.19
	azimuth	30° ± 34	−25° → 80°

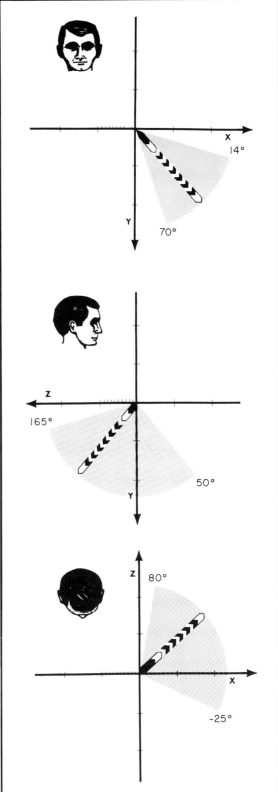

Fig. 1-157. Diagram to illustrate the 96 percent range of orientation of the maximal QRS vector in the frontal, right sagittal and horizontal plane.

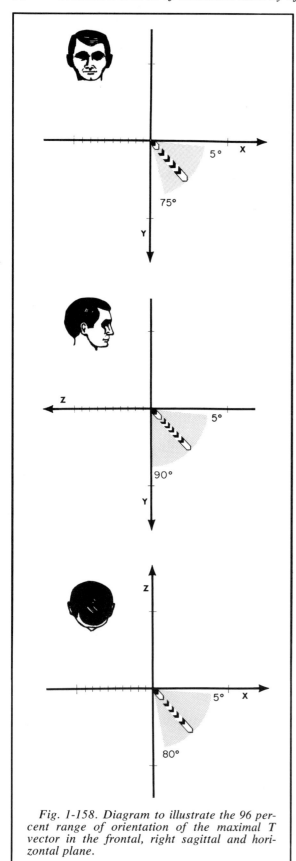

Fig. 1-158. Diagram to illustrate the 96 percent range of orientation of the maximal T vector in the frontal, right sagittal and horizontal plane.

TABLE 1-7. NORMAL VALUES OF THE MAXIMAL T VECTOR MAGNITUDE (IN MILLIVOLTS) AND ORIENTATION (IN DEGREES)

		MEAN ± SD	MIN → MAX
3-Dimen-sional Space	amplitude	0.46 ± 0.16	0.18 → 0.82
	azimuth	44° ± 19	4° → 79°
	elevation	29° ± 13	2° → 58°
Frontal Plane	amplitude	0.35 ± 0.14	0.12 → 0.70
	azimuth	40° ± 20	5° → 75°
Right Sagittal Plane	amplitude	0.35 ± 0.13	0.13 → 0.70
	azimuth	40° ± 20	5° → 90°
Hori-zontal Plane	amplitude	0.40 ± 0.15	0.15 → 0.75
	azimuth	45° ± 20	5° → 80°

Normal P Vector

X, Y, Z components. The spatial P vector can be visualized as the mean vector resulting from summation of two vectors: one representing the right atrium and the other representing the left atrium (Fig. 1-159). The vector of the right atrium is oriented anteriorly, downward and slightly to the left. The vector of the left atrium is oriented leftward, posteriorly and slightly upward. The resultant vector (i.e., the mean P vector), is oriented inferiorly, to the left, and slightly anteriorly or slightly posteriorly. The spatial P loop is normally oriented in the same direction as the mean P vector (Fig. 1-160). This loop may show a circular, oval or triangular shape and does not close because of the atrial depolarization.

The main characteristics of the normal X, Y, and Z components of the spatial P vector are shown in Figure 1-160. The P wave in the X lead is always positive, since the P vector is oriented to the left (i.e., it projects on the positive side of the X lead axis). The P wave in the Y lead is always positive, since the P vector is oriented inferiorly (i.e., it projects on the positive side of the Y lead axis). The P wave in the Z lead may be negative, biphasic (−+) or positive, since the P vector may be oriented either anteriorly, partially anteriorly and partially posteriorly, or posteriorly.

Each component can be resolved into a part representing the right atrial depolarization (vector) and a part representing the left atrial depolarization (vector), as shown in Figure 1-161. The depolarization of the right atrium corresponds to the ascending limb of the P wave, and the depolarization of the left atrium corresponds to the descending limb of the P wave. At the peak of the P wave, the activation of both atria is superimposed.

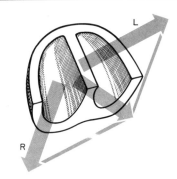

Fig. 1-159. Diagram to illustrate the formation of the mean P vector (as seen in the frontal plane).

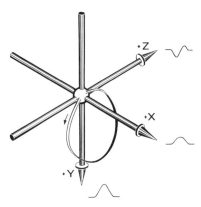

Fig. 1-160. Diagram showing the normal spatial P loop and its projections recorded in X, Y, and Z leads.

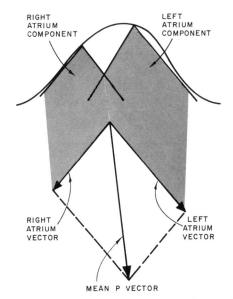

Fig. 1-161. Diagram to illustrate the resolution of the P vector (wave) into the right atrium and left atrium component.

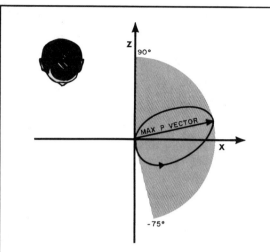

Fig. 1-162. Diagram showing the horizontal plane P loop.

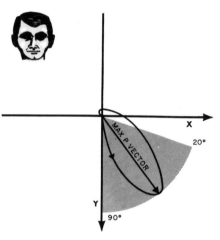

Fig. 1-163. Diagram showing the frontal plane P loop.

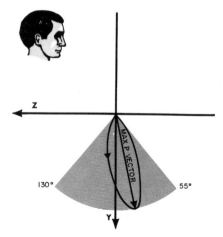

Fig. 1-164. Diagram showing the right sagittal plane P loop.

Planar projections. Planar projections of the spatial P loop have been studied very little, because much of the P loop is obscured by the initial and terminal parts of the T and QRS loops. However, this difficulty has been considerably overcome in recent vectorcardiographs.

A representative normal P loop in the horizontal plane is shown in Figure 1-162. It is usually very small, oval and shows counterclockwise rotation. The direction of the maximum P vector ranges from −75° to 90° with the mean of 10°. The magnitude of the maximum P vector is normally less than 0.2 mv.

A representative normal P loop in the frontal plane is shown in Figure 1-163. It is usually elongated and shows counterclockwise rotation. The direction of the maximum P vector ranges from 20° to 90° with the mean of 65°. The magnitude of the maximum P vector is usually below 0.25 mv.

A representative normal P loop in the sagittal plane is shown in Figure 1-164. It is usually elongated or triangular and shows clockwise rotation in the right sagittal plane, and counterclockwise rotation in the left sagittal plane. The direction of the maximum P vector in the right sagittal plane ranges from 55° to 130° with the mean of 80°. The magnitude of the maximum P vector rarely exceeds 0.2 mv.

Normal QRS Vector

X, Y, Z components. For descriptive purpose the spatial QRS loop is divided into the initial portion, the main body and the terminal portion. Except for the initial portion, the entire QRS loop is oriented inferiorly, to the left and posteriorly. Such an orientation is dictated by the fact that the mass of the left ventricle, which is located in the left infero-posterior octant of the chest, is so much greater than that of the right ventricle, that it contributes overwhelmingly to the normal vectorcardiogram (Fig. 1-165). The initial and terminal vectors vary considerably with the position of the heart. The initial vectors are oriented anteriorly to the right or left and either superiorly (in a vertical heart position), or inferiorly (in a horizontal heart position). The terminal vectors are oriented posteriorly, slightly to the left or right and either superiorly (in a horizontal heart position), or inferiorly (in a vertical heart position).

The main characteristics of X, Y, and Z components of the normal spatial QRS vector are shown in Figure 1-166. Because of the spatial orientation of the initial, main and terminal QRS vectors, the X lead records either a qR or qRs pattern, with a q wave approximately 0.02 second or less, or an Rs pattern or R wave. The Y lead records similar patterns but when the X lead shows a qR, the Y lead may show Rs or vice versa. The Z lead normally shows a qR pattern with a q wave approximately 0.03 sec. and 0.4 mv.

Time intervals are measured in the following way. As the beginning of a wave, the first deflection in any one of the three simultaneously recorded leads is used. As the end of a wave, the last deflection in any one of the leads is used (see page 159).

Horizontal plane. In the horizontal plane, the QRS loop can be oval-, elliptical- or triangle-shaped. It is usually 1½–3 times longer than it is wide. The horizontal plane QRS loop is always inscribed in a counterclockwise direction (to the left and posteriorly) without any crossover. The initial portion of the loop is usually directed to the right and anteriorly, although in some individuals (about 15 percent) it may be directed anteriorly and to the left. The initial or 20-msec. vector has magnitude between 0.15 and 0.75 mv (with the mean of 0.4 mv), and its orientation ranges from 0° to −120° (with the mean of −50°). The main body of the QRS loop is directed to the left and slightly posteriorly. The maximum QRS vector magnitude varies from 0.8 to 1.9 mv (with the mean of 1.3 mv), and its orientation ranges from −25° to 80° (with the mean of +10°). The terminal portion of the loop is usually directed posteriorly and slightly to the right or left. The terminal 20 msec. vector has magnitude between 0 and 0.9 mv (with the mean of 0.45 mv), and its orientation ranges from 125° to 35° with the mean of −90° (Fig. 1-167).

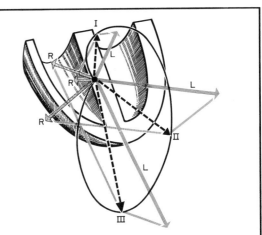

Fig. 1-165. Diagram to explain the fact that the left ventricle contributes overwhelmingly to the normal vectorcardiogram. For simplicity only 3 mean QRS vectors in the frontal plane are shown.

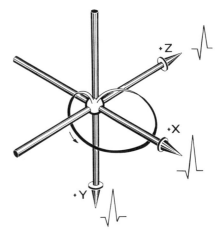

Fig. 1-166. Diagram showing the normal spatial QRS loop and its projections recorded in X, Y, and Z leads.

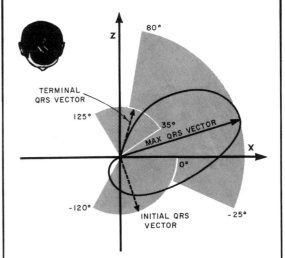

Fig. 1-167. Diagram showing the horizontal plane QRS loop.

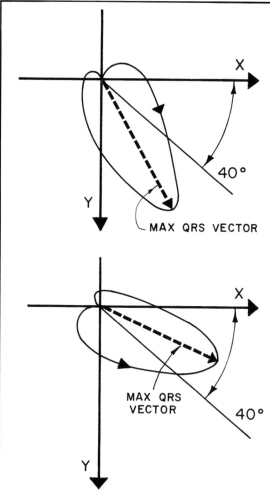

Fig. 1-168. *Diagram showing the relation between the direction of inscription of the QRS loop in the frontal plane and the orientation of the maximal QRS vector.*

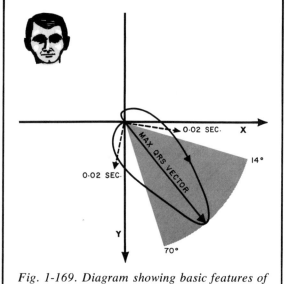

Fig. 1-169. *Diagram showing basic features of the frontal plane QRS loop.*

Frontal plane. In the frontal plane, most QRS loops are seen "on edge," because the spatial QRS loop is more or less perpendicular to this plane. Consequently, the frontal plane QRS loops are usually elongated and relatively narrow. The direction of the inscription of the loop is closely related to the position of the maximum QRS vector (Fig. 1-168). The QRS loop in the frontal plane is inscribed in a clockwise direction in those cases (about 65 percent), with the more vertically oriented maximum QRS vectors (lying above 40°). The QRS loop tends to be inscribed in a counterclockwise direction in these cases (about 10 percent), with more horizontally placed maximum QRS vectors (situated below 40°). In some normal individuals (about 25 percent) the QRS loop in the frontal plane displays a figure-of-eight pattern. The variable direction of inscription of QRS loop in the frontal plane is due to the fact that this loop is viewed nearly edge on and, therefore only a slight degree of rotation of the loop about its longitudinal axis causes a change in the apparent rotation.

The initial or 20 msec. vector has its magnitude between 0.05 and 0.7 mv (with the mean of 0.3 mv), and its orientation varies extremely, with a range covering the entire angular scale. However, when the frontal plane loop is clockwise, the initial forces must go beneath the E point by 0.02 sec. (or through E point by 0.016 sec.). The maximum QRS vector magnitude ranges from 1.0 to 2.2 mv (with the mean of 1.5 mv); its orientation varies from 14° to 70° with the average direction of 35°. The terminal 20 msec. vector has magnitude between 0 and 0.6 mv (with the mean of 0.25 mv) and its orientation is widely scattered, but usually it is directed inferiorly and to the right (Fig. 1-169).

Sagittal plane. In the sagittal plane the QRS loop may be oval-, elliptical- or triangle-shaped. In the left sagittal plane, the loop is inscribed in a counterclockwise direction, while in the right sagittal plane it is inscribed in a clockwise direction. There is, as yet, a lack of uniform recording of the sagittal plane; while the new recommendations of the

American Heart Association favor the recording in the left sagittal plane, most workers record the right sagittal plane vectorcardiograms; hence, such data are more common. The initial portion of the loop in the right sagittal plane is directed anteriorly and somewhat superiorly. The initial or 20-msec. vector has magnitude between 0.1 and 0.6 mv (with the mean of 0.3 mv) and its orientation varies from −30° to 75° (with the mean of 15°). The main body of the loop is directed inferiorly with most of the efferent limb situated anteriorly and most of the afferent limb situated posteriorly. The maximum QRS vector magnitude ranges from 0.3 to 1.9 mv (with the mean of about 1 mv). The direction of the maximum QRS vector ranges from 50° to 165° with the mean of 100°. The terminal 20 msec. vector has magnitude between 0.1 to 1.0 mv (with the mean of 0.5 mv) and its orientation ranges from 115° to −140°, with the mean of 160° (Fig. 1-170).

Normal ST Vector

The vector that extends from the origin of the QRS loop to its end or the beginning of the T loop (J point) is called the ST vector (Fig. 1-171). Such a vector occurs when the QRS loop fails to close (i.e., the inscription of the T loop starts before the QRS loop has returned to the isopotential line). The existence of this vector is manifested in X, Y, and Z leads by elevation or depression of the ST segment (Fig. 1-172). Usually, the ST segment rests on the isoelectrical line but slight elevation or depression can occur under normal conditions.

The magnitude of the ST vector is usually very small and does not exceed 0.1 mv in any planar projection, especially in older subjects. However, in children, a magnitude of 0.2 mv is still regarded as normal. The direction of the ST vector is concordant with the direction of the maximum T vector (i.e., the ST vector is oriented anteriorly and leftward in the horizontal plane, inferiorly and leftward in the frontal plane, and anteriorly and inferiorly in the right sagittal plane).

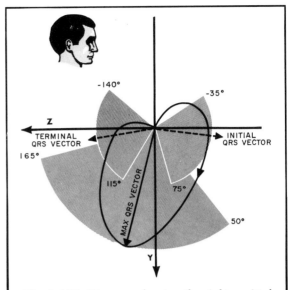

Fig. 1-170. Diagram showing the right sagittal plane QRS loop.

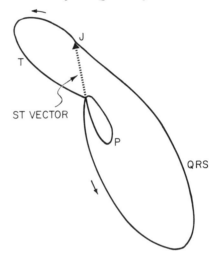

Fig. 1-171. Diagram to illustrate the formation of the ST vector.

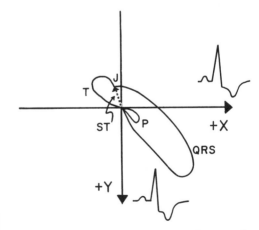

Fig. 1-172. Diagram to illustrate the recording of the ST vector in scalar leads.

Normal T Vector

X, Y, Z components. The spatial T loop is normally elongated or elliptical-shaped and its long axis is concordant with the long axis of the QRS loop (i.e., it is oriented anteriorly, inferiorly and to the left). The main characteristics of X, Y, Z components of the normal spatial T vector are shown in Figure 1-173. The X lead records an upward T, because the mean T vector projects on the left (or positive) side of the X lead axis. The Y lead records an upward, flat or slightly downward T wave, because the mean T vector projects on the inferior (or positive) side of the Y lead axis. The Z lead records negative T wave, because the mean T vector projects on the anterior (or negative) side of the Z lead axis. The initial limb of the T wave in any lead has a more gentle slope than the terminal limb, which either descends abruptly or rises rapidly to the base line.

Planar projections. The T loop in each plane is usually elongated and fusiform with a length-to-width ratio of 2.5 or greater. The direction of inscription of the T loop is usually concordant with that of the QRS loop (i.e., it is clockwise, when the QRS loop is inscribed clockwise, and vice versa). The speed of inscription of the T loop is not uniform—the initial portion of the T loop (or the efferent limb) is inscribed more slowly than the terminal portion (or the afferent limb); only abnormal T loops are uniformly inscribed. This area of normal delay is indicated by a closer lineup of the dashes (see page 60).

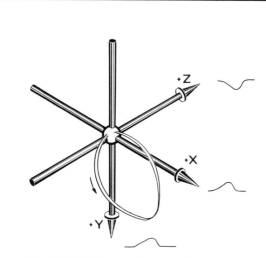

Fig. 1-173. Diagram showing the normal spatial T loop and its projections recorded in X, Y, and Z leads.

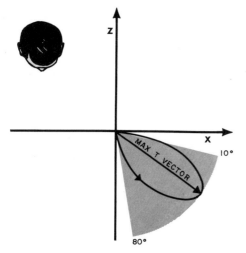

Fig. 1-174. Diagram showing the horizontal plane T loop.

In the horizontal plane, the T loop is inscribed in a counterclockwise direction, although in rare cases it may be inscribed clockwise or the direction of inscription cannot be determined because of the linear shape of the loop. The maximum T vector magnitude ranges from 0.25 to 0.75 mv with the mean of 0.50 mv. Orientation of the maximum T vector ranges from 10° to 80°, with the mean of 35° (Fig. 1-174).

In the frontal plane, the T loop can be inscribed either clockwise or counterclockwise. In some subjects the direction of inscription of the T loop may be opposite to that of the QRS loop. The maximum T vector magnitude ranges from 0.25 to 0.75 mv with the mean of 0.45 mv. Orientation of the maximum T vector ranges from 10° to 75°, with the mean of 35° (Fig. 1-175).

In the sagittal plane, the T loop is inscribed counterclockwise in the left sagittal view, and clockwise in the right sagittal view. The maximum T vector magnitude ranges from 0.2 to 0.7 mv with the mean of 0.4 mv. The orientation of the maximum T vector ranges from 10° to 90°, with the mean 45° in the right sagittal plane (Fig. 1-176). The angle between the maximum QRS and T vectors in normal subjects is quite variable and for this reason does not have much clinical value. Only in the frontal plane the angle is quite narrow and usually does not exceed 45°. However, in the horizontal and sagittal planes the QRS-T angle ranges from 25° to 150°.

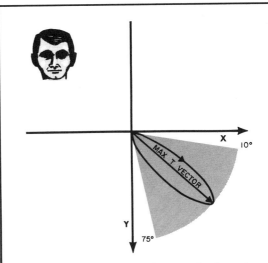

Fig. 1-175. Diagram showing the frontal plane T loop.

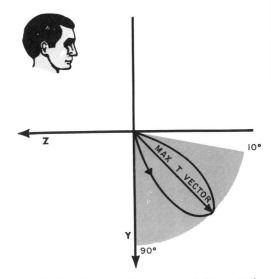

Fig. 1-176. Diagram showing the right sagittal plane T loop.

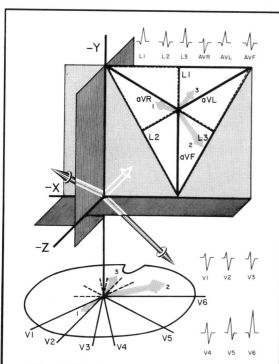

Fig. 1-177. Diagram to illustrate the frontal and horizontal plane initial (1) major (2) and terminal (3) QRS vectors and their projections on the 12 lead system's axes resulting in characteristic QRS configurations recorded in conventional electrocardiograms.

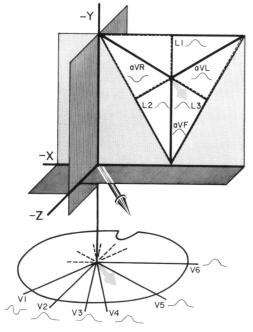

Fig. 1-178. Diagram to illustrate the frontal and horizontal plane mean P vectors and their projections on the 12 lead system's axes resulting in different polarity of the P wave recorded in conventional electrocardiograms.

NORMAL 12 LEAD ELECTROCARDIOGRAM

Genesis of the Normal ECG Pattern

The ECG pattern in any lead of the 12 lead system is a record of the potential variation against time. Further, the potential variation at a given moment during the cardiac cycle can be visualized as the projection of the instantaneous heart spatial vector on a given lead axis.

The relationship between the ECG pattern and the heart vector magnitude and orientation is illustrated in Figure 1-177. This figure depicts how the instantaneous vectors generated by ventricular depolarization may be grouped into three mean (or resultant) vectors, and how these vectors project on the lead axes. If a given vector projects onto the negative side of the lead axis, a negative deflection is recorded in this lead, and if this vector projects onto the positive side of the lead axis, a positive deflection is recorded in this lead.

All instantaneous vectors that are generated in the septum, within the first 10 to 15 msec. of depolarization, may be represented by a mean vector, called the initial QRS vector (in Fig. 1-177 this vector is designated by the number 1). In space this vector is directed anteriorly to the right and slightly inferiorly or superiorly depending upon the position of the heart. The most consistent feature is its anterior and rightward direction, which produces Q waves in lead L1 and in the leftward precordial leads, and small R waves in the rightward precordial leads. The orientation of the initial QRS vector in the supero-inferior direction is much less consistent and is related to the direction of the body of the QRS loop. In subjects in whom the mean QRS vector is horizontal, the initial QRS vector is usually directed inferiorly producing a Q wave in leads AVL. With a vertical mean QRS vector, the initial QRS vector is usually directed superiorly producing a Q wave in leads L2, L3, and AVF.

The major QRS vector results from all instantaneous vectors that are generated by the left ventricular free wall. (N.B.: Vectors representing electrical forces generated by the right ventricle are smaller and lag in time slightly more than those generated by the left ventricle. For this reason, the vector of the two ventricles combined is determined for the greater part by the left ventricle.) In space this vector is directed to the left, posteriorly and either inferiorly or superiorly depending on the position of the heart. The scalar components of this vector are recorded as positive deflections (R waves) in leads L1, L2, L3, and in the late precordial leads, or as negative deflections (S waves) in lead AVR and the rightward precordial leads. However, in the horizontal heart position the major QRS vector produces negative potential in lead L3, and in the vertical heart position this vector gives rise to negative potential in lead L1.

The terminal QRS vector results from all instantaneous vectors that are generated in the posterobasal part of the left ventricle and septum during the last 15 msec. of depolarization. In space this vector is oriented posteriorly, superiorly and slightly to the right. The scalar components of this vector are recorded as negative deflections (s waves) in leads L2, L3, and AVF, or as a positive deflection (terminal r or r¹ wave) in the rightward precordial leads.

It is apparent that the vectors corresponding to the Q or S deflections are oriented in the direction opposite to that giving rise to the R deflection. On the other hand, a vector which appears as a Q wave in one lead presents itself as an R wave in another lead. It depends on whether that vector projects onto the negative or positive side of the lead axis, and this is related in some extent to the position of the heart.

The successive instantaneous vectors generated during atrial depolarization also may be represented by a resultant (mean) P vector. In space the mean P vector is oriented to the left, inferiorly and slightly anteriorly or posteriorly. The scalar components of this vector are recorded as positive deflections (positive P wave) in leads L1, L2, L3, AVF, V4, V5, V6, or as negative deflections (inverted P wave) in lead AVR; leads AVL, V1, V2, and V3 record a positive P wave, biphasic P wave or inverted P wave (Fig. 1-178).

The successive instantaneous vectors generated during ventricular repolarization also may be represented by a resultant (mean) T vector. The orientation of this vector is usually, but not always, concordant with that of the major QRS vector. Thus it follows that the T wave polarity is usually concordant with that of the major QRS deflection. Normally, the T is always upright in leads L1, L2 and AVF, but may be positive, negative or diphasic in lead L3. It is always inverted in lead AVR. Its direction in lead AVL is dependent upon the electrical position. Thus, it is upright in the horizontal heart (when the QRS complex is positive), but may be inverted in vertical hearts (when the QRS complex is diphasic or negative). The polarity of the T wave in the precordial leads is usually positive, although it is not infrequently diphasic or inverted in V1 and V2 (Fig. 1-179).

Statistical Characteristics of the Normal ECG Data

Normal values of the 12 lead system electrocardiograms are listed in Tables 1-8 and 1-9. In particular cases many of these values represent cardiac abnormalities as well; therefore, they should be interpreted in the context of the entire tracing and in the light of clinical history and physical examination. Table 1-8 lists normal ranges (minimum → maximum) of amplitude measurements in mm in adults. Graphical representation of these normal ranges is shown in Figure 1-180. All time measurements in this figure are fictitious. Some of the descriptions and abbreviations used in Table 1-8 should be interpreted in the following way: "dominant" means the largest deflection in the QRS complex; "small q" means Q duration less than 0.04 sec. and Q amplitude less than 25 percent of the R amp.; "(A)" means depending on the electrical axis of the heart; "VHP" stands for the vertical heart position; "HHP" stands for the horizontal heart position.

Table 1-9 lists normal values of time measurements in adults. The PR interval is measured from the beginning of the P wave to the onset of the QRS complex. Both the PR interval and the P wave duration are usually measured in

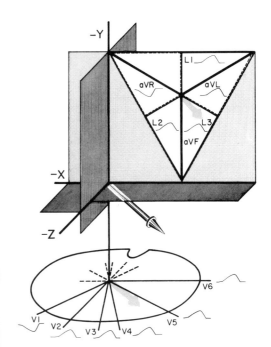

Fig. 1-179. Diagram to illustrate the frontal and horizontal plane mean T vectors and their projections on the 12 lead system's axes resulting in different polarity of the T wave recorded in conventional electrocardiograms.

TABLE 1-9.

P duration in lead L2	0.07	→ 0.13 sec.
PR interval in lead L2	0.10	→ 0.20 sec.
QRS interval	0.08	→ 0.11 sec.
Q duration	less than 0.04 sec.	
QR interval in V1	0.005	→ 0.03 sec.
QR interval in V6	0.02	→ 0.05 sec.
QT interval	0.30	→ 0.48 sec.

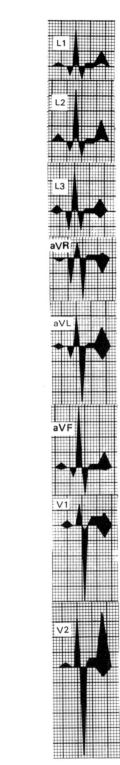

Fig. 1-180. Diagram to illustrate the 96 percent range of amplitude measurements (in mm) in the 12 lead system electrocardiograms.

lead L2. The QR interval is measured from the onset of the Q wave (or R wave if no Q wave is present) to the peak of the R wave. The QRS interval is measured from the onset of the Q wave (or R wave if no Q wave is present) to the

TABLE 1-8

	P	Q	R
Lead L1	positive 0.1 → 1.3	small 0.0 → 3.0	dominant 1.0 → 12.0
Lead L2	positive 0.3 → 2.5	small or none 0.0 → 3.0	dominant 2.0 → 17.0
Lead L3	variable −0.5 → 2.0	none, small or large (A) 0.0 → 6.0	none to dominant (A) 1.0 → 13.0
Lead aVR	negative −1.0 → 0.1	none, small or large; or QS pattern (A); 0.0 → 8.00	small or none (A) 0.0 → 5.0
Lead aVL	variable −0.5 → 0.8	small or none; large or QS pattern in VHP 0.0 → 3.5	small, none or dominant (A); 0.0 → 10.0
Lead aVF	positive −0.3 → 1.5	small or none 0.0 → 3.0	small, none or dominant (A); 0.0 → 20.0
Lead V1	variable −0.8 → 1.6	none or QS pattern 0.0 → 0.0	small or none; 0.0 → 7.0
Lead V2	variable −0.2 → 1.6	none or QS pattern 0.0 → 0.0	small or none 0.0 → 16.0
Lead V3	positive 0.0 → 1.8	small or none; 0.0 → 0.5	small, equal to S or dominant; 1.5 → 26.0
Lead V4	positive 0.1 → 2.3	small or none 0.0 → 1.6	small, equal to S or dominant 4.0 → 27.0
Lead V5	positive 0.0 → 2.4	small 0.0 → 2.1	dominant 4.0 → 26.0
Lead V6	positive 0.0 → 1.4	small 0.0 → 2.7	dominant 4.0 → 22.0

end of the S wave (or R wave if no S wave is present). The QT interval is measured from the onset of the Q wave (or R wave if no Q wave is present) to the end of the T wave.

TABLE 1-8

S	ST	T
small or none 0.0 → 4.0	isoelectric −0.5 → 1.0	positive 1.0 → 5.0
small or none 0.0 → 5.0	isoelectric −0.5 → 1.0	positive 1.0 → 7.0
none to dominant (A) 0.0 → 6.0	isoelectric −0.5 → 1.0	variable (A) −2.0 → 4.0
none or dominant; or QS pattern (A); 0.0 → 13.0	isoelectric −0.5 → 1.0	negative −5.0 → 1.5
none to dominant (A); 0.0 → 18.0	isoelectric −0.5 → 1.0	variable (A) −4.0 → 6.0
none or small; or dominant in HHP 0.0 → 8.0	isoelectric −0.5 → 1.0	variable (A) −0.5 → 5.0
dominant or QS pattern 2.0 → 25.0	slightly elevated 0.0 → 3.0	variable −4.0 → 4.0
dominant or QS pattern 0.0 → 29.0	slightly elevated 0.0 → 3.0	variable −3.0 → 18.0
dominant equal to R or small 0.0 → 25.0	slightly elevated 0.0 → 3.0	positive −2.0 → 16.0
small, equal to R or dominant 0.0 → 20.0	isoelectric −0.5 → 1.0	positive 0.0 → 17.00
small 0.0 → 6.0	isoelectric −0.5 → 1.0	positive 0.0 → 9.0
small 0.0 → 7.0	isoelectric −0.5 → 1.0	positive −0.5 → 5.0

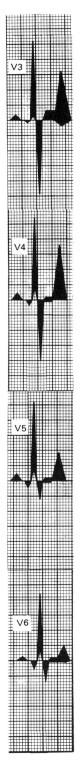

Fig. 1-180. Diagram to illustrate the 96 percent range of amplitude measurements (in mm.) in the 12 lead system electrocardiograms.

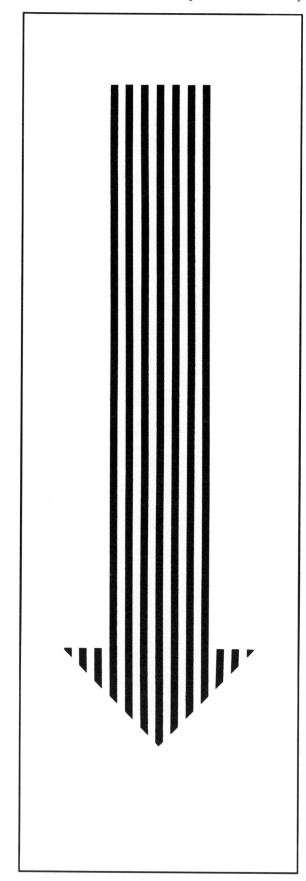

Abnormal Patterns of Electrical Activity of the Heart

GENERAL CONSIDERATIONS

Assessment of Abnormality

The first step in examining the vectorcardiogram is to make sure that the recording was made correctly (i.e., that the calibration and timing are right, and that the patient was breathing quietly during the recording). Deep inspiration causes QRS voltage reduction, which could mask the left ventricular hypertrophy; on the other hand, breath holding is followed by abnormal patterns resembling right ventricular hypertrophy.

In the process of diagnostic evaluation of the vectorcardiogram, the physician must first decide whether or not the VCG items are within normal limits. If they are, it is very likely (though not invariably) that the VCG comes from the normal subject. If the VCG items are outside normal limits, then the physician should try to answer the question of whether or not this could be due to physiological factors (i.e., constitutional variables, medication, smoking, etc.).

After excluding the possibility of the VCG being normal, the physician makes an hypothesis that it represents a certain abnormality. In many cases, abnormal findings in the vectorcardiogram can be interpreted with a fairly high degree of probability; they include ventricular conduction defects, recent myocardial infarction, old myocardial infarction, left ventricular hypertrophy, digitalis effect. More difficult to interpret are the minor abnormalities of the ST and T vectors which can be due to coronary insufficiency as well as to a variety of other factors (see page 130). Obviously, in this group of VCG abnormalities it is very easy to mistake a probably benign pattern as indicative of coronary artery disease. It is therefore advisable that the interpreter first consider the probability of normality.

As a rule, the diagnosis of the heart condition is based on a complete investigation, which includes the case history, auscultation and phonocardiogram, electrocardiogram and/or vectorcardiogram, X-ray examination, biochemical examination, and eventually catheterization and other methods. Thus, it is obvious that only the physician who is familiar with the patient and knows the results of all those examinations can arrive at a correct clinical diagnosis. On the other hand, any single diagnostic procedure does not provide sufficient information for a clinical diagnosis. However, this ideal requirement has been more or less violated in practice, since there is a natural tendency to make a quick diagnosis. This is especially true in the case of the electrocardiogram and/or vectorcardiogram where the physician expects from the interpreter an actual clinical diagnosis, such as myocardial infarction, ventricular hypertrophy, etc.

Classification of VCG Abnormalities

Individual differences between patients are so large that distinctive VCG patterns are recorded in almost each case. However, all abnormal vectorcardiograms can be classified into a few categories:

1. VCG tracings reflecting ventricular and/or atrial hypertrophy
2. VCG tracings reflecting ventricular conduction defects
3. VCG tracings reflecting myocardial infarction, injury or ischemia
4. VCG tracings displaying left axis deviation with no other abnormality
5. VCG tracings displaying nonspecific T vector changes.

Hypertrophy of one or the other ventricle results in a characteristic pattern of increased magnitude of QRS vectors, and in alteration of their direction; these are accompanied by the change in direction of T vectors (so-called secondary T vector changes).

Abnormal spread of depolarization, due to the blocking of the conduction pathway, alters the direction of the QRS vectors, slows their propagation and prolongs depolarization time. This is also accompanied by the change in direction of the T vectors (so-called secondary T vector changes).

Death of a region of the myocardium, being electrically inert, shifts the initial QRS vectors in an opposite direction to the site of the infarction. Depending on the stage of evolution of an infarction, QRS vectors may be accompanied by ST-T vector changes.

In some cases the only abnormality in the vectorcardiogram is the left axis deviation. Its significance is discussed on page 128.

Nonspecific T vector changes are said to be present if there is no abnormality in QRS vectors. Such changes are also called "primary, nonspecific T vector changes" as opposed to "secondary T vector changes," which are associated with the QRS vector abnormalities (hypertrophy, conduction defects, infarction). In each instance of "primary, nonspecific T vector changes," an etiologic factor can be traced only by examination of the associated clinical picture. Usually such changes are found in ischemia, myocarditis, digitalis intake, electrolyte disturbances (hypopotassemia, hyperpotassemia), metabolic and endocrine disturbances, and many other conditions.

Differentiation between primary and secondary T vector changes can be accomplished on mathematical grounds by means of the ventricular gradient concept (see page 27). Changes of the T vector associated with changes of the ventricular gradient are classified as primary T vector changes. Changes of the T vector at the constant ventricular gradient are classified as secondary T vector changes.

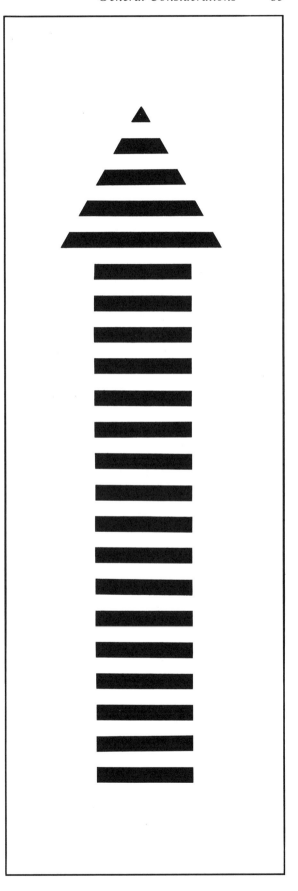

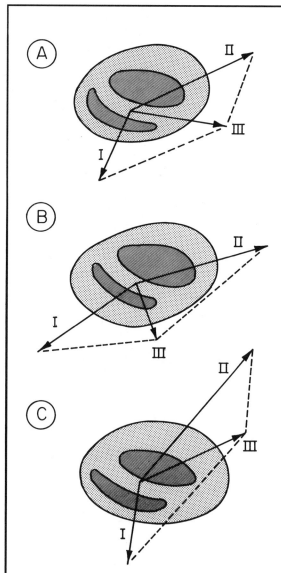

Fig. 1-181. Diagram to illustrate the resultant QRS vector when both ventricles are normal (top), when the right ventricle is hypertrophied (middle) and when the left ventricle is hypertrophied (bottom). Electrical forces produced by the right ventricle are designated by I, those produced by the left ventricle by II, and the resultant vector by III.

VECTOR INTERPRETATION OF VCG ABNORMALITIES

Pattern of Hypertrophy

Increased muscular mass of the heart (or hypertrophy), resulting from the excessive load on one part of the heart or the other, generates the depolarization vectors that are larger in magnitude. Another factor that may be responsible for the increased magnitude of the depolarization vectors is lessening of the distance between the hypertrophied chamber and the chest wall.

Increased magnitude of the depolarization vectors often tends to alter the direction of the mean vector (be it the mean P or QRS vector) toward the free wall of the hypertrophied chamber. When the right side chamber is involved, the mean depolarization vector shifts forward and usually to the right; when the left side chamber is involved, the mean depolarization vector shifts backward and usually to the left.

The principal vector changes occurring in hypertrophy of the cardiac chambers are illustrated in Figure 1-181. Figure 1-181 top depicts schematically the resultant vector (in the horizontal plane), as obtained by summing the vector representing forces generated by the normal right ventricular free wall, and the vector representing forces generated by the normal left ventricular free wall. This vector points anteriorly and to the left. Figure 1-181 middle depicts schematically the resultant vector, as obtained by summing the vector representing forces generated by the hypertrophied right ventricular free wall, and the vector representing forces generated by the normal left ventricular free wall. It is evident that this vector has been shifted anteriorly by the hypertrophied right ventricle.

The increased wall thickness, dilatation of the heart muscle, and possibly also the secondary changes (ischemia, fibrosis, etc.), affect the ventricular conduction system. This leads to some delay in the spread of activation and secondary disturbances of repolarization.

Pattern of a Ventricular Conduction Defect

Under physiologic conditions, both ventricles are activated almost simultaneously. When the impulse is blocked in one of the main divisions of the bundle of His, the sequence of ventricular depolarization is modified to a variable degree, and the vectorcardiogram demonstrates abnormal configurations, which are described as the left bundle branch block pattern (see page 104), and the right bundle branch block pattern (see page 107).

In addition, there is also a marked delay in the spread of depolarization manifested in the vectorcardiogram, by a closer lineup of the dashes making up the middle and/or terminal part of the QRS loop (Fig. 1-182). Localized slowing seen in only one plane is not sufficient evidence of true conduction delay, because this may be only a planar projection phenomenon. There should be slowing in at least two planes to be certain that slowed conduction actually exists.

When the spread of activation is delayed, the depolarization lasts longer than in the normal heart, thus resulting in an increased QRS loop duration. The total QRS duration is easily determined by counting the number of dashes making up the loop, and multiplying the total by the time interval between them. Bundle branch block is regarded as complete when the QRS loop lasts at least 0.12 sec., as incomplete when the QRS loop lasts shorter than 0.12 sec., but longer than 0.10 sec.

Since in bundle branch block the activation spreads along abnormal pathways, it follows that the regression of activation (or repolarization) is likewise pathological. As a purely secondary phenomenon there is usually a displacement of the ST and T vectors in the opposite direction to that of the QRS vectors (Fig. 1-183).

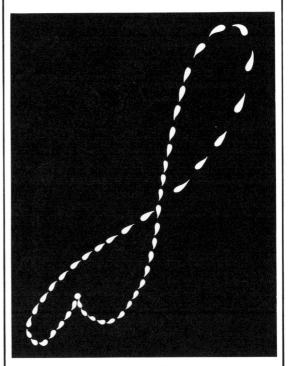

Fig. 1-182. Diagram to illustrate the slowing of inscription of the QRS loop and increased QRS loop duration. The duration of the QRS loop = 48 dashes × 0.0025 sec. = 0.120 sec.

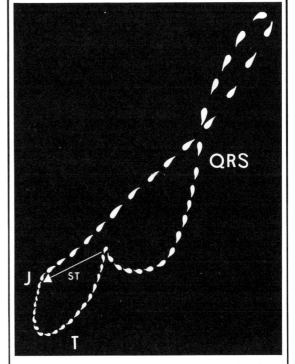

Fig. 1-183. Diagram to illustrate the displacement of the ST and T vectors in the opposite direction to that of the QRS vectors.

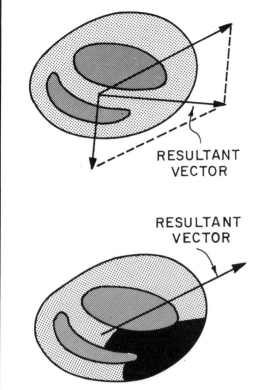

Fig. 1-184. *Diagram to illustrate shifting of the initial (0.04 sec.) QRS vector because the infarcted area is electrically inert. A) The 0.04 sec. QRS vector (as seen in the horizontal plane) in normal cases. B) The 0.04 sec. QRS vector (as seen in the horizontal plane) when the septal area is infarcted.*

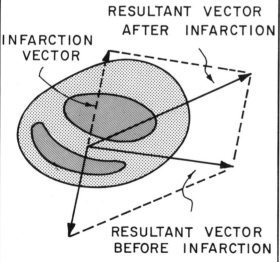

Fig. 1-185. *Diagram to illustrate the concept of the infarction vector (see text for details).*

Pattern of Myocardial Infarction

Myocardial infarction is caused by the necrosis of a localized area of the heart muscle becoming secondary to a deficient blood supply. This dead area may be considered electrically inert; since it does not produce any QRS vectors, the vectors generated by the normal wall become more prominent. This has been illustrated in Figure 1-184. It shows schematically the two mean QRS vectors for the first 0.04 second of ventricular depolarization: one represents electrical forces generated by the septum, and another represents electrical forces generated by the free left ventricular wall. By summing these two vectors, the resultant vector for the first 0.04 second of ventricular depolarization is obtained. (N.B.: The free right ventricular wall vector has not been considered since its contribution to the resultant QRS vector is negligible.) This vector is directed anteriorly and to the left in the horizontal projection. Figure 1-184b shows what happens when the septal area is infarcted and does not generate electrical forces. In such a case, the resultant vector of the first 0.04 second of ventricular depolarization is determined only by the free left ventricle wall forces, which are represented by the mean vector pointed posteriorly and to the left when viewed in the horizontal plane.

Another vectorial interpretation of the myocardial infarction pattern involves subtracting the preinfarction vector from the postinfarction vector (Fig. 1-185). The vector which is obtained by such an operation is called an "infarction vector," and it represents the hypothetical electrical forces that are equal in magnitude but opposite in direction to those normally generated by the area before it became infarcted.

Thus, the absence of QRS vectors previously present in the infarcted area is directly responsible for the fact that QRS vectors generated elsewhere in the myocardium become representative of the whole myocardium. Consequently, the postinfarction resultant vector tends to point away from the side of the infarcted area. Thus, in anterior infarction the resultant vector is shifted posteriorly, and in posterior infarction the resultant vector is shifted anteriorly.

Change of the QRS vectors' direction influences the direction of the QRS loop inscription. Thus, the counterclockwise rotation, characteristic of the normal QRS loops in the horizontal and left sagittal plane may be replaced by partial or complete clockwise rotation.

The QRS vector changes occur only when the infarcted area has become completely dead, and they usually take place a few hours after an infarction. The change that develops immediately after an infarction and may last from a few hours up to two weeks is a current (or vector) of injury.

This vector originates at the site of an injured myocardial area as the result of two factors:

1. Partial or complete blocking of the depolarization wave at the borders of the region of injury;
2. Partial depolarization of the region of injury during the whole cardiac cycle.

At the completion of depolarization, the injured region (where the depolarization wave has been completely or partially blocked) retains a few positive charges and becomes positively charged, with respect to completely depolarized adjacent parts of the heart, thus acting as a dipole. This dipole can be represented by a vector directed away from the uninjured muscle and toward the injured area (Fig. 1-186). Thus, for example, a subepicardial injury of the anterior wall produces an injury vector oriented anteriorly, while a subendocardial injury of the same region produces an injury vector oriented posteriorly. Transmural myocardial infarction produces an injury vector similar to that of the subepicardial injury.

Another characteristic feature of a myocardial infarction is manifested by the T vector changes. They may begin to develop after a period of hours or days and may remain for many months or years. These changes are due to an area of ischemia which is adjacent to the area of injury.

Ischemia of the heart muscle causes a delay in the onset of the repolarization process of the ventricles. A consequence of this delay depends on the localization of ischemia. When ischemia occurs in the subendocardial layer of the heart muscle, it delays the repolarization process of this region but does not change the normal direction of repolarization, which is from the epicardium to the endocardium. Thus, the ischemic subendocardial muscle continues to repolarize for a time after opposing repolarization potentials from other regions have begun to subside. Consequently, the late instantaneous T vectors point away from the ischemic area and their magnitude is increased (Fig. 1-187A).

When ischemia occurs in the subepicardial layer of the heart muscle, a delay of the onset of repolarization of this region makes the endocardial muscle fibers depolarize first. The repolarization process is reversed, since it proceeds from the endocardium to the epicardium. In such a case, T vectors are directed in an epicardium-to-endocardium direction (i.e., they point away from the ischemic area, Fig. 1-187B). (N.B.: The T vector representing repolarization is opposite to the direction of the sequence of repolarization. For details see page 60.) Consequently, subepicardial ischemia of the anterior wall is manifested by T vectors oriented posteriorly, while that of the inferior wall is manifested by T vectors oriented superiorly. Transmural ischemia produces T vectors similar to those of the subepicardial ischemia.

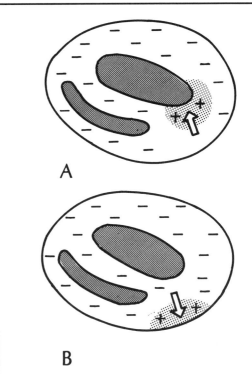

Fig. 1-186. Diagram to illustrate the direction of the injury vector in (A) subendocardial and (B) subepicardial infarction.

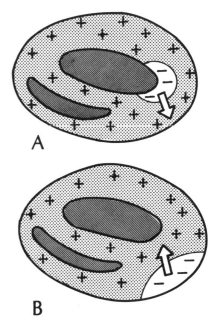

Fig. 1-187. Diagram to illustrate the direction of the T vector in (A) subendocardial and (B) subepicardial infarction.

Part 2
Vectorcardiogram in
Cardiac Disease

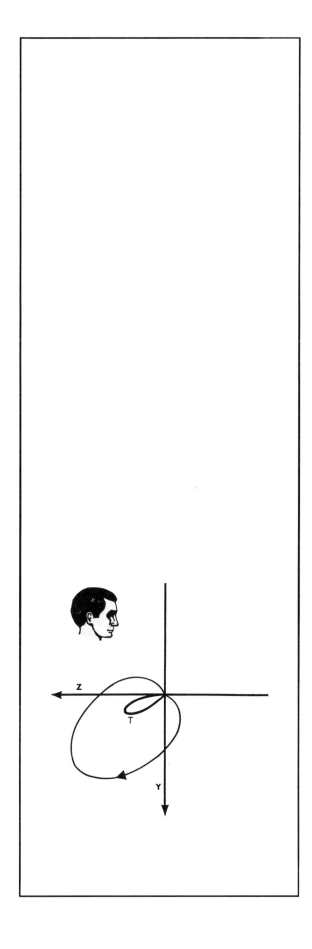

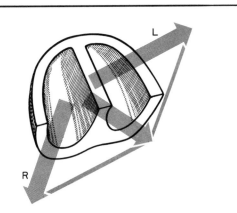

Fig. 2-1. Diagram depicting the mean P vector in the case of normal atria (as seen in the frontal plane).

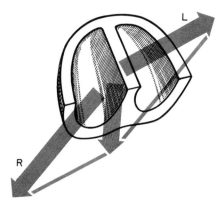

Fig. 2-2. Diagram depicting the mean P vector in right atrial enlargement (as seen in the frontal plane).

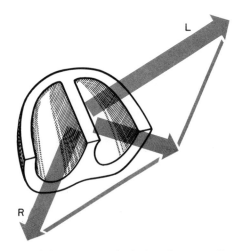

Fig. 2-3. Diagram depicting the mean P vector in left atrial enlargement (as seen in the frontal plane).

Hypertrophy of the Heart Muscle

VCG IN ATRIAL ENLARGEMENT

Origin and Occurrence

The VCG pattern of atrial enlargement is determined by the increased electrical forces of the hypertrophied left atrium, or right atrium or both atria.

When both atria are normal, the vectorial summation of the vector of the right atrium (which is directed anteriorly, inferiorly and slightly to the left) and the vector of the left atrium (which is directed to the left, posteriorly and slightly superiorly) gives rise to the resultant (or mean) P vector which is directed anteriorly, inferiorly and to the left (Fig. 2-1).

When the right atrium enlarges, its vectors of increased magnitude and anterior orientation are superimposed upon those from the left atrium, producing the mean P vector, which has an increased magnitude, and is oriented more anteriorly than normally (Fig. 2-2). The VCG pattern of right atrial enlargement is encountered most commonly in chronic cor pulmonale, tricuspid atresia, pulmonary stenosis, tetralogy of Fallot, interatrial septal defect, and persistent truncus arteriosus.

When the left atrium enlarges, its vectors of increased magnitude and posterior orientation are superimposed on the PQ segment, producing the mean P vector, which has only slightly increased magnitude and is oriented more posteriorly than normally (Fig. 2-3). The VCG pattern of left atrial enlargement is encountered most commonly in mitral stenosis and/or insufficiency, aortic valvular disease, hypertensive heart disease, interventricular septal defect, and constrictive pericarditis.

Usually the P loop is widely opened giving rise to an abnormally large atrial repolarization (T_a) vector which extends from the beginning to the end of the P loop and is oriented opposite to the direction of the maximum P vector.

Combined atrial (biatrial) enlargement produces VCG patterns that represent a variable combination of signs of right and left atrial enlargement.

Right Atrial Enlargement

Scalar X, Y, Z components. The spatial P loop in right atrial enlargement is abnormally large and displaced inferiorly, anteriorly and slightly to the left. The inferiorly oriented P vectors project on the positive side of the Y lead axis, giving rise to a P wave, whose amplitude exceeds 0.25 mv in this lead (Fig. 2-4).

Horizontal plane VCG. The P loop is elongated or egg-shaped and practically all of its area is located anteriorly. The direction of inscription is counterclockwise as in normal cases. The maximum P vector is oriented more anteriorly than normally, and its magnitude may be increased (Fig. 2-5).

Right sagittal plane VCG. The P loop is elongated or banana-shaped and inscribed in a clockwise direction, as in normal cases. The maximum P vector is oriented inferiorly and anteriorly and its magnitude exceeds 0.20 mv, which is the upper limit of normal (Fig. 2-5).

Frontal plane VCG. The P loop is elongated or pendulous-shaped and inscribed in a counterclockwise direction in most cases. The maximum P vector is oriented inferiorly and slightly to the left and its magnitude exceeds 0.20 mv, which is the upper limit of normal (Fig. 2-5).

Standard 12 lead electrocardiogram. The inferiorly oriented P vectors project on the positive side of the axis of lead L2, L3, and aVF, giving rise to a P wave of amplitude > 0.25 mv (often called the "P pulmonale") in these leads (Fig. 2-6).

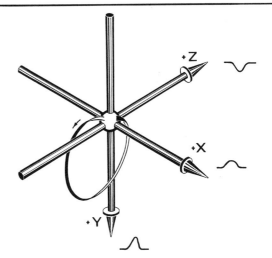

Fig. 2-4. Diagram showing the spatial P loop and its projections recorded in X, Y, and Z leads in right atrial enlargement.

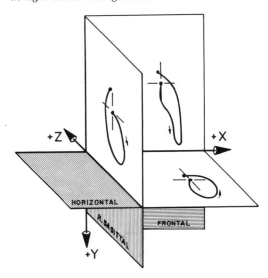

Fig. 2-5. Diagram of the horizontal, right sagittal and frontal plane P loop in right atrial enlargement.

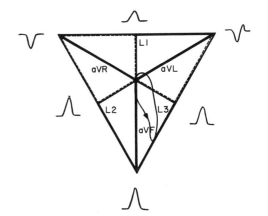

Fig. 2-6. Diagram depicting the P wave in limb leads in right atrial enlargement.

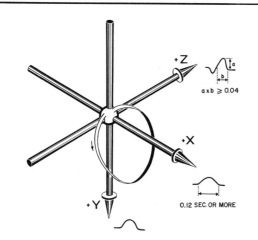

Fig. 2-7. *Diagram showing the spatial P loop and its projections recorded in X, Y, and Z leads in left atrial enlargement.*

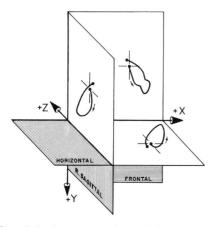

Fig. 2-8. *Diagram of the horizontal, right sagittal and frontal plane P loop in left atrial enlargement.*

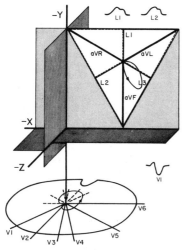

Fig. 2-9. *Diagram depicting the P wave in limb leads and precordial leads in left atrial enlargement.*

Left Atrial Enlargement

Scalar X, Y, Z components. The spatial P loop in left atrial enlargement is larger than normal and displaced posteriorly, inferiorly and to the left. The posteriorly oriented P vectors project on the positive side of the lead Z axis, giving rise to a monophasic upright P wave or a biphasic (−+) P wave, with a positive component of increased amplitude and/or duration (Fig. 2-7).

Horizontal plane VCG. The majority of the P loop is located in a posterior left quadrant. The direction of inscription is counterclockwise, or the loop displays a figure-of-eight pattern with the early portion inscribed counterclockwise. The maximum P vector is oriented posteriorly and to the left and its magnitude exceeds 0.10 mv, which is the upper limit of normal. In most cases the duration of the P loop is between 0.11 and 0.13 sec. (Fig. 2-8).

Right sagittal plane VCG. The P loop is located mainly in the posterior-inferior quadrant. The direction of inscription is clockwise, although a figure-of-eight pattern is not unusual (Fig. 2-8).

Frontal plane VCG. The P loop displays an irregular contour, due to one or more big notches. The direction of inscription is counterclockwise, although a figure-of-eight pattern may be seen occasionally. The maximum P vector is oriented more to the left than normally (Fig. 2-8).

Standard 12 lead electrocardiogram. The P vectors, oriented posteriorly and to the left, project on the negative side of the V1 lead axis and on the positive side of the lead L1 and L2 axis. Consequently, a negative P or a biphasic (+−) P wave with a negative component of increased amplitude and/or duration is recorded in lead V1, while a broad and notched P wave (so-called the "P mitrale") is recorded in lead L1 and L2 (Fig. 2-9).

VCG IN LEFT VENTRICULAR HYPERTROPHY

Origin and Occurrence

The VCG pattern of left ventricular hypertrophy results from the following anatomical changes: (1) increased muscle mass of the left ventricle; (2) lessening of the distance between the left ventricle and the chest wall; (3) positioning of the whole heart more horizontally (Fig. 2-10). The hypertrophied and somewhat dislocated left ventricle generates the vectors, which are not only larger but are also displaced farther posteriorly and to the left, as compared with the normal heart.

Increased intraventricular pressure usually results in ischemia of the subendocardial layer of the left ventricle. This ischemia by itself, or eventually together with metabolic changes in hypertrophied heart muscle, gives rise to ST and T vectors displaced to the right.

Left ventricular hypertrophy usually results from hypertensive heart disease, aortic valvular disease (aortic stenosis and/or aortic insufficiency), mitral insufficiency and some congenital heart diseases (patent ductus arteriosus, aortic or subaortic stenosis, ventricular septal defect, tricuspid atresia, coarctation of the aorta).

Scalar X, Y, Z Components

In most patients with left ventricular hypertrophy, the spatial QRS loop has increased magnitude and its body is located in the left, posterior and usually inferior octant of a three-dimensional space. The initial QRS vector is displaced to the left, slightly anteriorly and inferiorly. The terminal QRS vector is oriented to the left, posteriorly, and superiorly or inferiorly (Fig. 2-11). QRS vectors which are oriented to the left and posteriorly project on the positive side of the X and Z lead axes, giving rise to a tall R wave in these leads. Usually, at least in one of these leads, R amplitude is greater than 1.5 mv and the sum of R amp. in X and R amp. in Z is greater than 2.2 mv. In lead Z the R wave may be preceded by a small q wave which is caused by the initial QRS vector pointing anteriorly (Fig. 2-11).

The spatial T loop is displaced anteriorly, to the right and superiorly (i.e., in an opposite direction to that of the QRS loop). Frequently the T loop is open, giving rise to the ST vector whose magnitude is increased and the direction is parallel to the direction of the T loop. These ST-T vector changes are seen in X, Y, and Z leads as the ST segment and T wave pointing in a direction opposite to that of the main deflection of the QRS complex. The T wave is usually asymmetrical: the downstroke has a gradual slope, while the upstroke has a much steeper slope. When associated coronary heart disease is present the T wave may be symmetrical (see page 131).

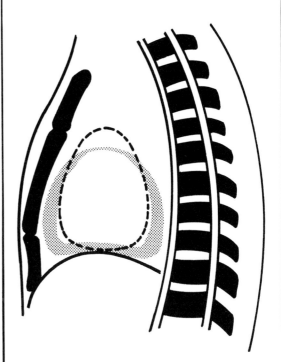

Fig. 2-10. Diagram showing the anatomical changes giving rise to the VCG pattern of left ventricular hypertrophy (as viewed from the left shoulder).

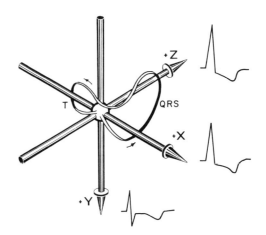

Fig. 2-11. Diagram showing the spatial QRS-T loop and its projections recorded in X, Y, and Z leads in left ventricular hypertrophy.

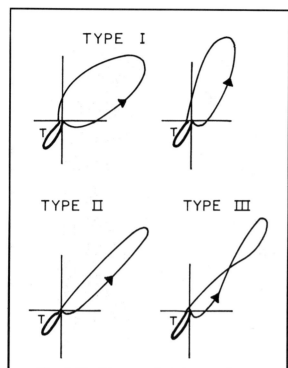

Fig. 2-12. Diagram depicting configuration and the direction of inscription of the horizontal plane QRS loop in left ventricular hypertrophy.

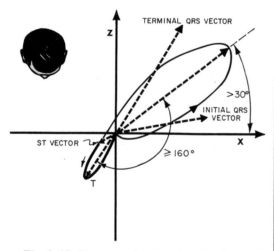

Fig. 2-13. Diagram showing the direction and magnitude of initial, maximal and terminal QRS vectors in the horizontal plane in left ventricular hypertrophy. The range of direction is indicated by the shadowed area.

Vectorcardiographic Loops

Characteristic features of left ventricular hypertrophy (i.e., the leftward and posterior displacement of the body and terminal vectors), are seen in all three planes because each of them involves either the X lead, or the Z lead or both.

Horizontal plane loop. 1. QRS loop configuration and direction of inscription. Usually the QRS loop is oval (type I) or elongated and narrow (type II) and inscribed counterclockwise. In cases of severe hypertrophy the loop presents a figure-of-eight configuration (type III) with the distal portion inscribed clockwise (Fig. 2-12). The body of the QRS loop is directed posteriorly and leftward. The duration of the QRS loop is often slightly prolonged (up to 0.11 sec.).

2. Direction and magnitude of the maximum QRS vector. The magnitude of the maximum QRS vector is greater than 2.2 mv below the age of 50 years and greater than 1.8 mv at the age of 50 years or more. The direction of this vector is usually displaced to +30° or more posteriorly (Fig. 2-13). Its time occurrence (after the beginning of the QRS loop) is sometimes prolonged (0.05 sec. or more).

3. Direction of the initial and terminal QRS vectors. Initial vectors normally oriented anteriorly and to the right are often reduced or replaced by vectors directed anteriorly and to the left. Terminal vectors normally directed posteriorly and to the right are replaced by vectors directed posteriorly and to the left (Fig. 2-13).

4. Morphology of the T loop. The long axis of the T loop is frequently directed to the right and anteriorly (i.e., in an opposite direction to that of the QRS long axis). This produces an abnormally wide QRS-T angle of 160° or more (Fig. 2-13). The T loop directed to the right and posteriorly is believed to reflect significant coronary sclerosis in association with LVH.

5. The ST vector. The magnitude of the ST vector is often increased because the QRS loop remains widely open. The direction of this vector is parallel to the direction of the T loop (Fig. 2-13).

Frontal plane loop. The entire QRS loop is frequently inscribed counterclockwise and is often wider than normal. The maximum QRS vector usually exceeds 2 mv and is directed to the left and downward or rarely upward. Initial QRS vectors are usually directed to the left and inferiorly or rarely to the right and superiorly (as in normal subjects). The T loop is displaced to the right and superiorly producing a wide QRS-T angle. The ST vector is parallel to the T loop (Fig. 2-14).

Right sagittal plane loop. The QRS loop is usually inscribed clockwise and has greater area than in normal cases. The maximum QRS vector often exceeds 2 mv and is directed posteriorly and inferiorly. Initial vectors are displaced downward and anteriorly. The T loop is displaced anteriorly moving opposite to the backwardly located QRS loop. The ST vector is parallel to the T loop (Fig. 2-15).

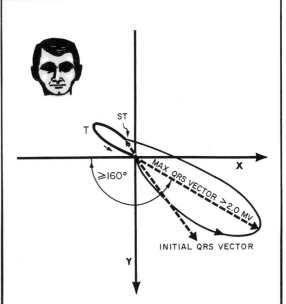

Fig. 2-14. Diagram of the frontal plane VCG in left ventricular hypertrophy.

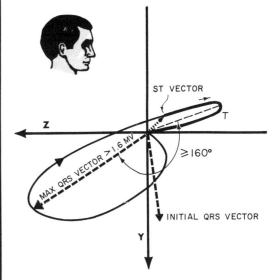

Fig. 2-15. Diagram of the right sagittal plane VCG in left ventricular hypertrophy.

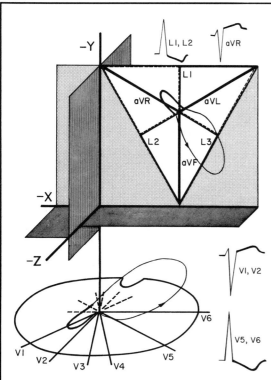

Fig. 2-16. Diagram of the 12 lead system electrocardiograms in left ventricular hypertrophy.

Standard 12 Lead ECG

QRS vectors which are oriented to the left and posteriorly in LVH, project on the positive side of the axis of leads L1, L2, and left precordial, giving rise to a tall R wave, a depressed ST segment, an inverted T wave with a slowly descending efferent limb and a rapidly ascending afferent limb. However, in L3, aVR and right precordial leads an rS pattern with a deep S wave or a QS complex is recorded as the QRS vectors project on the negative axis of these leads (Fig. 2-16).

VCG IN RIGHT VENTRICULAR HYPERTROPHY

Origin and Occurrence

The VCG pattern of right ventricular hypertrophy is determined by the increased electrical forces of the hypertrophied right ventricular muscle, which abolish the normal preponderance of the left ventricular forces. Thus, in right ventricular hypertrophy, QRS vectors are predominantly oriented to the right and anteriorly or posteriorly, depending on the hemodynamic mechanism causing the hypertrophy.

In order to reach this point a considerable degree of hypertrophy must be present since the left ventricle has 3 times as many muscle fibers as the right ventricle. Thus, at the early stage of RVH, the only diagnostic feature in the VCG is a forward displacement of the QRS vectors, which gives rise to a deep Q wave in lead Z (or a large R wave in lead V1) and the horizontal plane loop with at least 70 percent of its area being located anteriorly.

It is believed that the right ventricle becomes hypertrophied either due to pressure (systolic) overloading, or to volume (diastolic) overloading. Pressure overloading (i.e., an increase in the mean arterial pressure) as seen, for example, in mitral or pulmonary stenosis, leads to hypertrophy of the entire musculature of the right ventricle thus producing QRS vectors predominantly oriented to the right and anteriorly (Fig. 2-17A).

Volume overloading (i.e., an increase in the volume of blood per beat) as seen, for example, in atrial septal defect, leads to the localized hypertrophy of the basal right septal muscle and crista supraventricularis, producing QRS vectors predominantly oriented to the right and posteriorly (Fig. 2-17B). Although, in many instances this correlation does not apply; nevertheless, it is convenient to divide all VCG patterns of RVH into dextro-anterior and dextro-posterior type.

The pattern of RVH is normal in newborns up to the age 2 months and in some cases it can persist through childhood until adolescence (so-called juvenile pattern). It is encountered most often in patients with congenital heart disease (atrial septal defect, pulmonary stenosis, tetralogy of Fallot, Eisenmenger's complex, transposition of great vessels), mitral stenosis, chronic cor pulmonale, and pulmonary embolism.

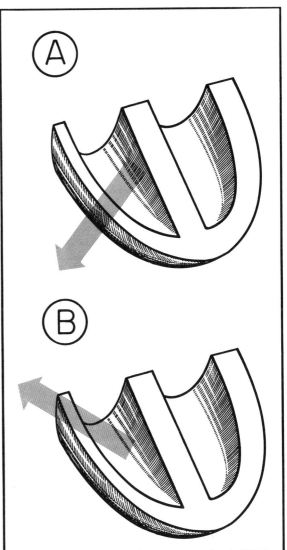

Fig. 2-17. Diagram depicting two basic VCG patterns of right ventricular hypertrophy (RVH) as seen in the horizontal plane. A. Dextro-anterior type of RVH due to pressure overloading. B. Dextro-posterior type of RVH due to volume overloading.

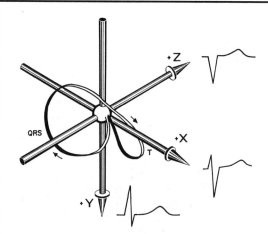

Fig. 2-18. Diagram showing the spatial QRS-T loop and its projections recorded in X, Y, and Z leads in dextro-anterior type of RVH.

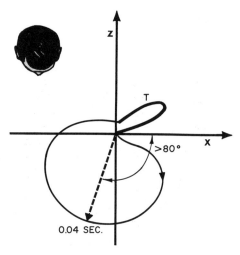

Fig. 2-19. Diagram of the horizontal plane VCG in dextro-anterior type of RVH.

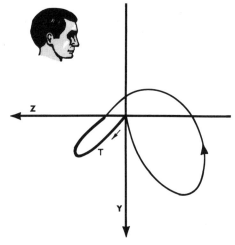

Fig. 2-20. Diagram of the right sagittal plane VCG in dextro-anterior type of RVH.

Dextro-Anterior Type of RVH

Scalar X, Y, Z components. This type of right ventricular hypertrophy pattern, which may be related to systolic overloading, is characterized by the spatial QRS loop, whose body and terminal portion are displaced to the right, anteriorly and either inferiorly or superiorly. Only the initial portion of the loop and the early efferent limb may be oriented to the left and anteriorly or posteriorly (Fig. 2-18).

The main and terminal QRS vectors displaced to the right and anteriorly, project on the negative side of the X and Y lead axes. Thus lead X displays an rS or RS pattern with a deep S wave resulting in an S/R ratio of 1.1 or more, while lead Z displays a QS complex or a Qr pattern with a deep Q wave (Fig. 2-18). In some cases all QRS vectors project on the negative side of the X lead axis giving rise to a QS pattern. The sum of anterior and rightward forces (i.e., an amplitude of the S wave in lead X plus amplitude of the Q wave in lead Z) is equal to or greater than 1.4 mv.

The spatial T loop is usually discordant to the terminal QRS vectors (i.e., oriented to the left, posteriorly and inferiorly). The ST vector, if present, is oriented in the same direction as the T loop.

Horizontal plane VCG. 1. QRS loop configuration and direction of inscription. Configuration of the QRS loop is variable, but in most cases the majority of the loop is located anteriorly and to the right. The direction of inscription is usually clockwise; however the loop may show a figure-of-eight configuration with the efferent limb inscribed counterclockwise. In mild cases of RVH, the rotation of the loop may remain normal (i.e., counterclockwise, Fig. 2-19).

2. Direction of the maximum QRS vector. The maximum or 0.04 sec. QRS vector is displaced rightward and anteriorly, the degree of this displacement being roughly proportionate to the degree of right ventricular hypertrophy. This vector is usually located between +80° and +130° (Fig. 2-19).

3. Direction of the initial and terminal QRS vectors. The initial portion of the QRS loop may start to move normally

(i.e., anteriorly and to the left), however, in most cases it moves anteriorly and to the right. The terminal portion of the loop may display normal direction or may be directed more anteriorly and to the right than normally (Fig. 2-19).

Right sagittal plane VCG. The QRS loop may show numerous configurations, depending on the degree of hypertrophy and the position of the heart. The direction of inscription is usually counterclockwise, but in some cases the loop may display a clockwise rotation or a figure-of-eight pattern. The initial portion and the body of the QRS loop are oriented anteriorly and inferiorly. The terminal portion is usually displaced superiorly and to the right. The T loop tends to swing posteriorly, and inferiorly or superiorly, principally opposite the terminal QRS vectors (Fig. 2-20).

Frontal plane VCG. The QRS loop is usually wide and inscribed in a clockwise direction. There is a characteristic bulging of the afferent limb of the loop, which gives rise to abnormally large terminal vectors pointing rightward and superiorly or inferiorly. The mean QRS vector is usually located in the +90° to +180° quadrant. The T loop is inscribed opposite the terminal QRS vector (Fig. 2-21).

Standard 12 lead electrocardiogram. The majority of the QRS vectors which in right ventricular hypertrophy are oriented to the right and anteriorly, project predominantly on the positive side of the axis of the right precordial leads and aVR, giving rise to a tall R wave or rSR′ pattern. In some cases a qR pattern may be seen if the initial QRS vectors are oriented to the left and posteriorly. The ST segment is slightly depressed and the T wave is inverted (with a slowly descending efferent limb and a rapidly ascending afferent limb) due to the abnormal posterior orientation of the ST and T vectors.

The left precordial leads, aVL, L1, and occasionally also L2 and L3 record rS or RS pattern, since the QRS vectors project predominantly on the negative side of the axis of these leads. The ST segment may be slightly elevated and the T wave is usually upright (Fig. 2-22).

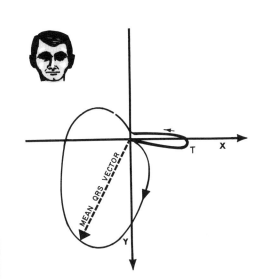

Fig. 2-21. Diagram of the frontal plane VCG in dextro-anterior type of RVH.

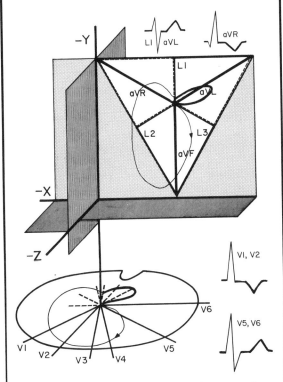

Fig. 2-22. Diagram of the 12 lead system electrocardiograms in dextro-anterior type of RVH.

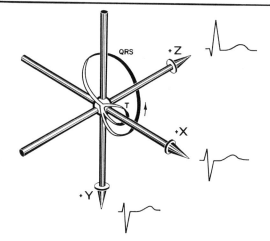

Fig. 2-23. Diagram showing the spatial QRS-T loop and its projections recorded in X, Y, and Z leads in dextro-posterior type of RVH.

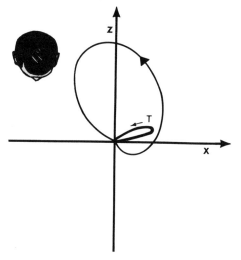

Fig. 2-24. Diagram of the horizontal plane VCG in dextro-posterior type of RVH.

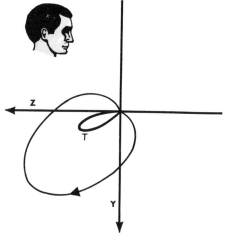

Fig. 2-25. Diagram of the right sagittal plane VCG in dextro-posterior type of RVH.

Dextro-Posterior Type of RVH

Scalar X, Y, Z components. This type of right ventricular hypertrophy pattern, which may be related to diastolic overloading of the right ventricle, is characterized by the spatial QRS loop, whose terminal portion and frequently the body are displaced to the right, posteriorly and either inferiorly or superiorly. The initial portion of the loop and the early efferent limb may be oriented to the left and anteriorly or posteriorly (Fig. 2-23).

The main and/or terminal QRS vector displaced to the right and posteriorly, project on the negative side of the X lead axis and on the positive side of the Z lead axis. Thus, lead X displays an rS or RS pattern with a deep S wave resulting in an S/R ratio of 1.1 or more, while lead Z records a tall R wave or a qR pattern (Fig. 2-23).

The spatial T loop is usually normal (i.e., oriented to the left, posteriorly or anteriorly and inferiorly).

Horizontal plane VCG. The QRS loop is located more posteriorly and to the right than in normal cases (i.e., more than 20 percent of the total QRS loop area is situated in the right posterior quadrant). The direction of inscription of the QRS loop is counterclockwise in most cases. However, a figure-of-eight pattern with a second half inscribed clockwise may be seen occasionally. The initial portion and sometimes, also, the early efferent limb, retain the normal orientation, while the rest of the loop is displaced to the right and posteriorly. The T loop is usually oriented to the left and posteriorly or anteriorly (Fig. 2-24).

Right sagittal plane VCG. The majority of the QRS loop is situated in the posterior and inferior quadrant. However, a considerable portion of the late afferent limb may be situated in the posterior and superior quadrant. The direction of inscription of the loop is variable but usually it is inscribed clockwise. The T loop is usually oriented inferiorly and posteriorly or sometimes anteriorly (Fig. 2-25).

Frontal plane VCG. The QRS loop is located more to the right of the midline (Y lead axis) than in normal cases, and in most cases exhibits a right superior bulging of the late afferent limb. Usually it shows a clockwise inscription. The T loop is oriented inferiorly and to the left (Fig. 2-26).

Standard 12 lead electrocardiogram. The main and terminal QRS vectors displaced to the right and posteriorly, project on the negative side of the axis of lead L1, aVL, right and midprecordial leads, and occasionally also leads L2, L3 and aVF. Consequently an rS pattern in these leads is usually recorded. However, in lead V1 a QS complex, or rSR′ pattern, may be seen occasionally.

The posterior orientation of the T loop gives rise to inverted T waves in the right precordial leads. The ST segment is usually within normal limits (Fig. 2-27).

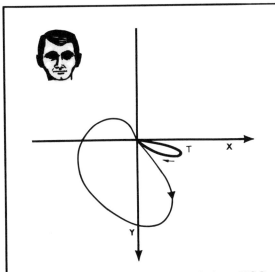

Fig. 2-26. *Diagram of the frontal plane VCG in dextro-posterior type of RVH.*

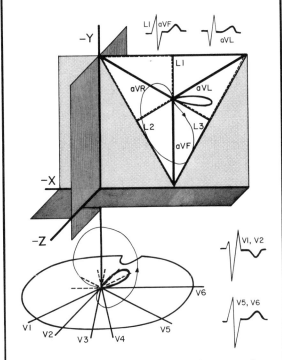

Fig. 2-27. *Diagram of the 12 lead system electrocardiograms in dextro-posterior type of RVH.*

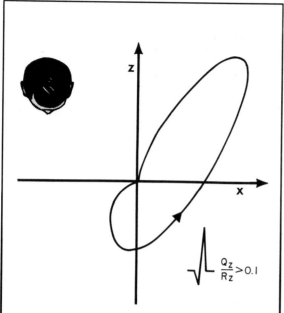

Fig. 2-28. *Diagram of the biventricular hypertrophy VCG in the horizontal plane showing the pattern of LVH associated with a marked anterior displacement of the early QRS vectors.*

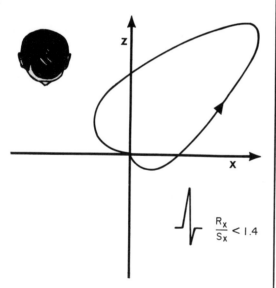

Fig. 2-29. *Diagram of the biventricular hypertrophy VCG in the horizontal plane showing the pattern of LVH associated with a marked rightward displacement of the late QRS vectors.*

VCG IN BIVENTRICULAR HYPERTROPHY

Origin and Occurrence

The vectorcardiographic diagnosis of biventricular hypertrophy is usually difficult. The lacking of diagnostic abnormalities in the VCG is due mainly to the following reasons:

1. A simultaneous hypertrophy of both ventricles may lead to a pseudo-normalization of the vectorcardiogram because QRS vectors displaced to the left and right cancel each other.

2. The more marked hypertrophy of the left ventricle is likely to produce only the VCG pattern of LVH.

3. The more marked hypertrophy of the right ventricle is likely to produce only the VCG pattern of RVH alone.

Only in a small number of cases the VCG shows, simultaneously, signs of both left and right ventricular hypertrophy. Usually the pattern of LVH predominates with only moderate evidence of RVH.

The VCG pattern of BVH is usually seen in mitral stenosis and/or mitral insufficiency, chronic pulmonary diseases, hypertensive heart disease, arteriosclerotic heart disease, aortic stenosis and/or aortic insufficiency, primary myocardial disease, and some congenital heart diseases (ventricular septal defect with pulmonary hypertension, patent ductus arteriosus with pulmonary hypertension, ostium primum defect, Ebstein's disease).

Diagnostic Features

The diagnosis of biventricular hypertrophy should be considered if one of the following features is seen in the VCG:

1. A marked anterior displacement of the QRS vectors in the presence of the VCG pattern of LVH. In such a case the horizontal plane QRS loop displays an anterior bulging and consequently the Q/R amplitude ratio in lead Z is greater than 0.1 and the R wave greater than 0.5 mv is recorded in the right precordial leads (Fig. 2-28).

2. A marked posterior displacement of the QRS vectors in the presence of the VCG pattern of LVH. In such a case the horizontal plane QRS loop displays a right posterior bulging, and consequently the R/S amplitude ratio in lead X is less than 1.4, and a deep S wave is recorded in leads L1, and the mid and left precordial leads (Fig. 2-29).

3. Right atrial enlargement in the presence of the VCG pattern of LVH (see page 93).

4. A marked left posterior displacement of the QRS vectors in the presence of the VCG pattern of RVH. In such a case the horizontal plane QRS loop is more or less isodiphasic in relation to the X and/or Z axes, the sum of R amplitude in lead X and R amplitude in lead Z is equal to or greater than 1.5 mv, and an RS pattern is recorded in most of the precordial leads (Fig. 2-30).

5. Left atrial enlargement in the presence of the VCG pattern of RVH (see page 97).

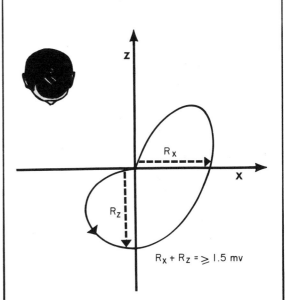

Fig. 2-30. Diagram of the biventricular hypertrophy VCG in the horizontal plane showing the pattern of RVH associated with a marked posterior displacement of the mid QRS vectors.

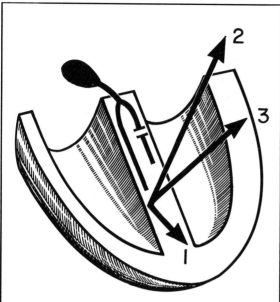

Fig. 2-31. Diagram showing the distorted sequence of ventricular depolarization in left bundle branch block (LBBB). The break in the conducting path is indicated by the double line across the left bundle branch.

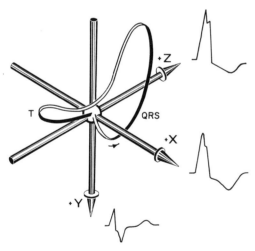

Fig. 2-32. Diagram showing the spatial QRS-T loop and its projections recorded in X, Y, and Z leads in LBBB.

Ventricular Conduction Defects

VCG IN LEFT BUNDLE BRANCH BLOCK

Origin and Occurrence

Left bundle branch block arises as a result either of complete or of partial impairment of conduction in the left branch of the bundle of His (Fig. 2-31). Although this impairment may occur in the anatomical sense, in many cases it represents a pathophysiological condition.

When the conduction down the left bundle is blocked, the activation proceeds down the right bundle branch so that the first part to undergo depolarization is the right septum and the free wall of the right ventricle. Consequently, the initial vector is oriented to the left, anteriorly and inferiorly. The activation of the left part of the septum proceeds in the right-to-left direction, thus giving rise to a vector directed to the left, posteriorly and inferiorly. The last part to undergo depolarization is the lateral wall of the left ventricle, which gives rise to a vector directed to the left, posteriorly and superiorly in relation to the previous vector (Fig. 2-31).

The VCG pattern of LBBB is rarely encountered in otherwise healthy subjects; it is usually associated with one of the following clinical conditions: coronary insufficiency, infarction, left ventricular hypertrophy (hypertension, aortic valve disease), mitral stenosis, congenital septal defect, some infectious diseases (diphtheria, bacterial endocarditis, etc.), and some drug intoxications (quinidine, digitalis, procainamide).

Scalar X, Y, Z Components

The spatial QRS loop in left bundle branch block is elongated, narrow, and oriented posteriorly, leftward and either slightly inferiorly or superiorly. The initial portion, however, may be inscribed anteriorly, leftward and inferiorly (Fig. 2-32).

The accentuated posterior and leftward orientation of the spatial QRS loop is reflected by a tall, wide and slurred R wave in leads X and Z. This indicates that all instantaneous QRS vectors point on the positive (i.e., posterior in lead Z and leftward in lead X) side of the axis of a particular lead (Fig. 2-32). Occasionally, when the initial portion of the QRS loop is inscribed anteriorly the Z lead shows a qR pattern, with a small q wave. When the QRS duration is greater than 0.12 sec. the left bundle branch block is regarded as complete; when the QRS duration is 0.11 to 0.12 sec., the left bundle branch block is incomplete.

The QRS loop is open, giving rise to the ST vector, which is oriented anteriorly and to the right (i.e., in an opposite direction to that of the QRS loop). The T loop is oriented in the same direction as the ST vector.

Vectorcardiographic Loops

Characteristic findings of LBBB (i.e., the posterior and leftward displacement of the entire QRS loop) are seen in all three planes, because each of them involves either the X lead, or Z lead or both.

Horizontal plane. The QRS loop is elongated and considerably narrow. The initial 0.01 sec. QRS vector is directed anteriorly and leftward and moves in a counterclockwise direction. The body of the QRS loop is oriented posteriorly and to the left and inscribed in a clockwise direction. In some cases there may be a crossover at the apex or base of the loop, giving rise to a figure-of-eight configuration. The slowing of conduction, as indicated by closely spaced dots, usually starts at the midportion of the QRS loop and involves the rest of the loop. The total QRS duration is thus increased to 0.12 sec. or more. The maximum QRS vector often exceeds 2 mv and is located in the left posterior quadrant within the range from −50° to −85°.

The QRS loop usually does not return to the isoelectric point, there being the ST vector which is oriented to the right and anteriorly. The T loop is oriented opposite to the QRS loop giving rise to a wide QRS-T angle measuring about 180° (Fig. 2-33).

Right sagittal plane. The initial 0.001 sec. QRS vector is usually oriented anteriorly and inferiorly and moves in a counterclockwise direction. The body of the loop is oriented posteriorly and inscribed in a clockwise direction. The slowing of conduction, as indicated by closely spaced dots, usually involves the mid and terminal portions of the loop. The total QRS duration is thus increased to 0.12 sec. or more. The maximum QRS vector has increased magnitude and is directed posteriorly within the range from 150° to 180°. The ST vector and the T loop are oriented opposite to the QRS loop (Fig. 2-34).

Frontal plane. The whole body of the QRS loop is located on the left side and inscribed in a counterclockwise direction. There is slowing of the mid and terminal portions of the QRS loop. The maximum QRS vector usually has normal or decreased magnitude and tends to assume a horizontal position, the usual range being from −15° to 50°. The ST vector and the T loop are oriented opposite to the QRS loop (Fig. 2-35).

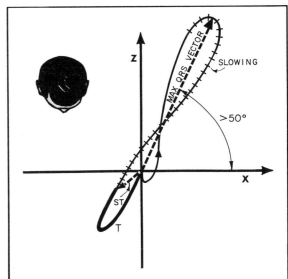

Fig. 2-33. Diagram of the horizontal plane VCG in LBBB.

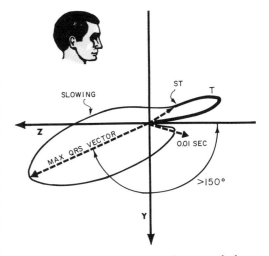

Fig. 2-34. Diagram of the right sagittal plane VCG in LBBB.

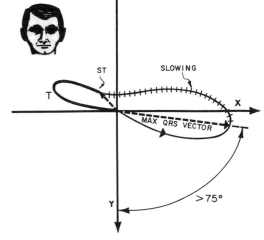

Fig. 2-35. Diagram of the frontal plane VCG in LBBB.

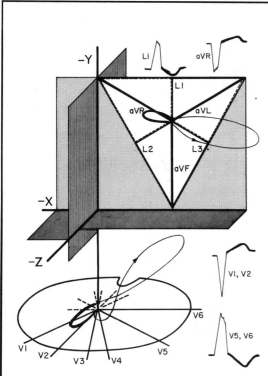

Fig. 2-36. Diagram of the 12 lead system electrocardiograms in LBBB.

Standard 12 Lead Electrocardiogram

The QRS vectors which are oriented posteriorly and to the left in LBBB, project on the negative side of the axis of the right precordial leads, and on the positive side of the axis of the left precordial leads and L1. Consequently, a QS complex is recorded in leads V1-V3 and a tall, slurred R wave with no preceding q wave in V5-V6 and L1. In many instances, however, instead of the QS complex an rS pattern is recorded in V1-V3; a small but consistent r wave in these leads reflects the initial 0.01 QRS vector being projected on the positive side of the right precordial lead axis. The ST segment and the T wave are discordant to the QRS complex (i.e., the ST segment is depressed and the T wave is negative in L1, V5-V6) while in leads V1-V2 there is an elevated ST segment and an upright T wave (Fig. 2-36).

VCG IN RIGHT BUNDLE BRANCH BLOCK

Origin and Occurrence

Right bundle branch block arises as a result of either complete or partial impairment of conduction in the right branch of the bundle of His (Fig. 2-37). Although this impairment occurs in the anatomical sense, in many cases it represents a pathophysiological condition.

When the conduction down the right bundle is blocked, the activation of the left part of the septum and the left ventricle is normal; however, the activation of the right part of the septum and the right ventricle spreads along muscular pathways from the left side, when the depolarization of the free wall of the left ventricle is almost complete. Subsequently, vectors representing unopposed depolarization of the right ventricle are not only delayed but also are directed to the right and anteriorly (Fig. 2-37).

The VCG pattern of incomplete RBBB is frequently encountered in otherwise healthy subjects, especially the young. In most cases, however, complete RBBB is associated with one of the following clinical conditions: coronary artery disease, hypertensive heart disease, right ventricular hypertrophy, congenital septal defects, some infectious diseases (diphtheria, bacterial endocarditis, etc.), and some drug intoxications (quinidine, digitalis, procainamide).

Scalar X, Y, Z Components

The spatial QRS loop in right bundle branch block differs from the normal in that the terminal vectors representing abnormal depolarization of the right septum and the free wall of the right ventricle form a finger-like appendage, which is oriented to the right and anteriorly. The initial and body vectors are in a more or less normal position in the uncomplicated RBBB (Fig. 2-38).

The rightward and anterior displacements of the terminal QRS vectors are reflected by a qRS pattern with a wide and slurred S wave in lead X and Z, indicating that these vectors project on the negative side (i.e., rightward in lead X and anterior in lead Z) of a corresponding lead axis (Fig. 2-38). When the QRS duration is equal to or greater than 0.12 sec. right bundle branch block is regarded as complete; when the QRS duration is 0.10 to 0.11 sec. right bundle branch block is incomplete.

The QRS loop may be open, thus giving rise to the ST vector which is usually small and directed to the left and posteriorly (i.e., in an opposite direction to that of the terminal QRS vector). The T loop is oriented in the same direction as the ST vector.

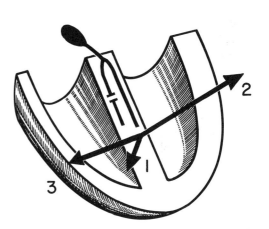

Fig. 2-37. Diagram showing ventricular depolarization vectors in the case of right bundle branch block (RBBB). The break in the conducting path is indicated by the double line across the right bundle branch.

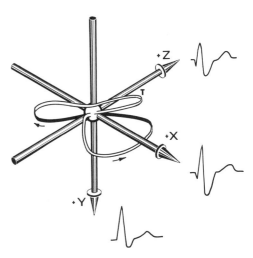

Fig. 2-38. Diagram showing the spatial QRS-T loop and its projections recorded in X, Y, and Z leads in RBBB.

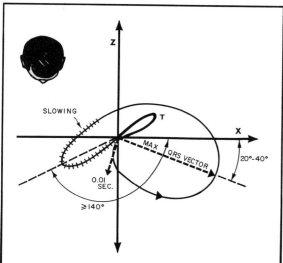

Fig. 2-39. Diagram of the horizontal plane VCG in RBBB.

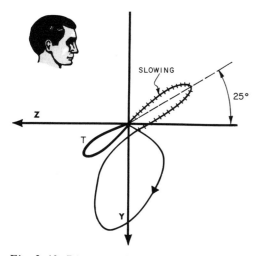

Fig. 2-40. Diagram of the right sagittal plane VCG in RBBB.

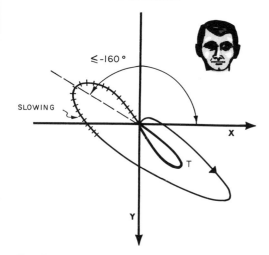

Fig. 2-41. Diagram of the frontal plane VCG in RBBB.

Vectorcardiographic Loops

Characteristic findings of RBBB (i.e., the rightward and anterior displacement of the terminal QRS vectors) are seen in all three planes, because each of them involves either the X lead, or Z lead or both.

Horizontal plane loop. The initial QRS vector is oriented normally (i.e., anteriorly and to the right). Also, the efferent limb of the loop has a normal appearance (i.e., it points to the left and anteriorly and is inscribed in a counterclockwise direction). However, the afferent limb is usually displaced anteriorly and in some cases it may cross over the efferent limb (resulting in a figure-of-eight pattern), or it may become entirely anterior to the efferent limb so that most of the QRS loop is inscribed clockwise. The duration of the QRS loop is prolonged to 0.12 sec. or more.

The terminal QRS vectors are directed to the right and anteriorly and from a finger-like appendage whose average direction is 140°. Most of this appendage is slowly inscribed, as indicated by close spacing between dots.

The maximum QRS vector is smaller and its orientation is more anterior as compared with normal QRS loops. In uncomplicated RBBB the maximum QRS vector is usually located between 20° and 40°. When this vector is at −20° or less, one may consider the coincident presence of left ventricular hypertrophy. When RBBB is complicated by right ventricular hypertrophy, the maximum QRS vector is usually oriented at 90° or more.

The T loop is oriented to the left and posteriorly (i.e., in an opposite direction to the terminal appendage of the QRS loop). The ST vector is usually very small or not present (Fig. 2-39).

Right sagittal plane. The initial QRS vectors are normally oriented (i.e., anteriorly and inferiorly). The main

QRS vectors may retain normal (i.e., anterior-inferior) direction and clockwise inscription, or they may be oriented superiorly and posteriorly, and inscribed counterclockwise or partially counterclockwise (figure-of-eight pattern). The terminal QRS vectors are usually oriented anteriorly and superiorly and form an appendage whose average direction is −25°. These vectors are slowly inscribed, as indicated by close spacing between dots. The T loop is directed in an opposite direction to that of the terminal QRS vectors (Fig. 2-40).

Frontal plane loop. The orientation of the initial and main QRS vectors is quite variable. The terminal QRS vectors are oriented to the right and superiorly, the average direction being −160°. They are slowly inscribed, as indicated by close spacing between dots. The direction of inscription may be clockwise or counterclockwise, the latter being almost always associated with a wide and superiorly oriented QRS loop. Leftward and superior displacement of the QRS loop producing left axis deviation generally indicates the coincident presence of left ventricular hypertrophy. The T loop is oriented in an opposite direction to that of the terminal QRS vectors (Fig. 2-41).

Standard 12 Lead Electrocardiogram

The terminal QRS vectors oriented anteriorly and to the right in RBBB, project on the negative side of the axis of the left precordial leads and leads L1, L2 and sometimes L3, giving rise to a wide and slurred S wave in these leads. Lead V1 and sometimes V2 record an RSR' pattern because the terminal QRS vectors point on the positive side of the axis of the right precordial leads. The T wave is usually discordant to the terminal component of the QRS complex (i.e., it is positive when a wide S is recorded and negative when a broad R' is recorded, Fig. 2-42).

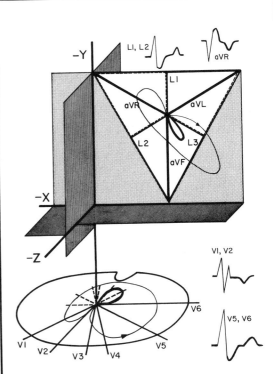

Fig. 2-42. Diagram of the 12 lead system electrocardiograms in RBBB.

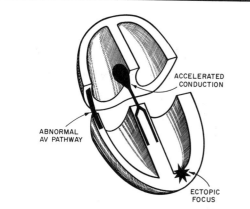

Fig. 2-43. Diagram depicting a possible mechanism underlying the WPW syndrome.

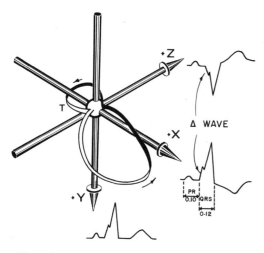

Fig. 2-44. Diagram showing the spatial QRS-T loop and its projections recorded in X, Y, and Z leads in type A WPWS.

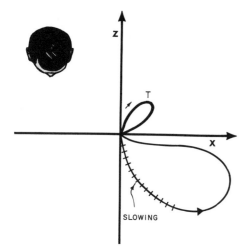

Fig. 2-45. Diagram of the horizontal plane VCG in type A WPWS.

VCG IN THE WOLFF-PARKINSON-WHITE SYNDROME

Origin and Occurrence

The exact mechanism of Wolff-Parkinson-White, or ventricular preexcitation, syndrome has not yet been completely clarified. However, it is a generally accepted idea that premature depolarization affects only a segment of the ventricular myocardium, while the remaining ventricular muscle is activated in the usual manner. This phenomenon is ascribed to one of the following causes: (1) the presence of abnormal atrioventricular muscular bundle; (2) the existence of an ectopic ventricular focus that is activated either electrically or mechanically from the atria (implying localized inflammatory or degenerative injury of the heart muscle); (3) accelerated conduction by way of normal AV node (Fig. 2-43). The syndrome has been separated into type A, believed to be caused by premature activation of the left ventricle, and type B caused by premature activation of the right ventricle.

In general, the WPW syndrome is of no clinical significance, although, frequently, it is accompanied by attacks of paroxysmal supraventricular tachycardia. The syndrome is observed frequently in certain congenital cardiac malformations, especially in the Ebstein's anomaly. Patients with coronary artery disease, thyrotoxicosis, and hypertrophic subaortic stenosis seem to have a higher incidence of this syndrome in comparison with those who do not have these problems.

Type A WPW Syndrome

Scalar X, Y, Z components. The principal alteration of the spatial QRS loop in type A WPW syndrome is a slowing of the initial portion of the loop which runs anteriorly, leftward and usually inferiorly, as does the remainder of the loop (Fig. 2-44). Since the initial QRS vector projects on the positive side of the X lead axis, a small upward deflection (so-called delta wave), marking the onset of the R wave, is recorded in this lead. The anterior orientation of the initial QRS vector implies that this vector projects on the negative side of the Z lead axis, thus a small downward deflection (delta wave), marking the onset of the Q wave or QS complex, is recorded in lead Z. Presence of the delta wave accounts for a widening of the QRS complex (0.11 to 0.14 sec.) at the expense of the PR interval. Thus, in lead X and Z the PR interval measures only 0.10 sec. or less (Fig. 2-44).

Horizontal plane loop. The initial QRS vector is oriented always anteriorly and usually to the left but occasionally to the right. The maximum QRS vector is oriented anteriorly and to the left. The QRS loop is usually inscribed in a counterclockwise direction, although a figure-of-eight pattern may be recorded occasionally. The initial portion of the QRS loop and sometimes almost the entire efferent limb displays conduction delay as indicated by close spacing between dots. The T loop may be opposite to the QRS loop (Fig. 2-45).

Right sagittal plane loop. The initial QRS vector is directed anteriorly and inferiorly in most instances. The body of the QRS loop is invariably located anteriorly and inferiorly (or superiorly). The direction of inscription of the QRS loop is usually clockwise, however, a figure-of-eight pattern may be recorded occasionally (Fig. 2-46).

Frontal plane loop. The QRS loop configuration and inscription is quite variable. The initial QRS vectors are slowly inscribed and usually point to the left and either inferiorly or superiorly (Fig. 2-47). One must be careful not to overlook the initial slowing which is the most important factor in proper assessment of the superiorly oriented initial QRS vectors, which otherwise could be interpreted as a pattern of an inferior myocardial infarction.

Standard 12 lead electrocardiograms. The QRS vectors oriented anteriorly and to the left, project on the positive side of the axis of left and right precordial leads and almost all limb leads (except aVR lead), giving rise to a large R wave with an initial upward deflection (delta wave) in these leads (Fig. 2-48). The PR interval is 0.10 sec. or less.

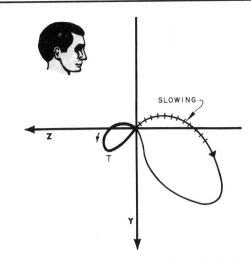

Fig. 2-46. Diagram of the right sagittal plane VCG in type A WPWS.

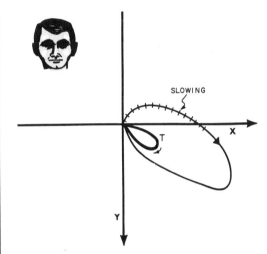

Fig. 2-47. Diagram of the frontal plane VCG in type A WPWS.

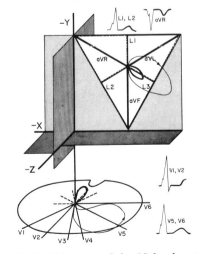

Fig. 2-48. Diagram of the 12 lead system electrocardiograms in type A WPWS.

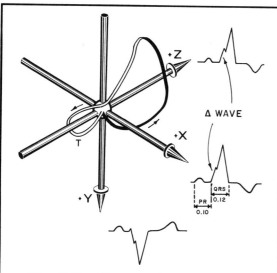

Fig. 2-49. *Diagram showing the spatial QRS-T loop and its projections recorded in X, Y, and Z leads in type B WPWS.*

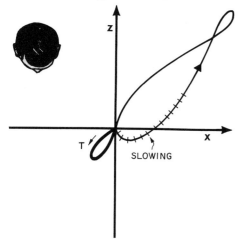

Fig. 2-50. *Diagram of the horizontal plane VCG in type B WPWS.*

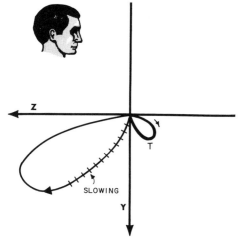

Fig. 2-51. *Diagram of the right sagittal plane VCG in type B WPWS.*

Type B WPW Syndrome

Scalar X, Y, Z components. The principal alteration of the spatial QRS loop in type B WPW syndrome is a slowing of the initial portion of the loop which may start anteriorly but run chiefly posteriorly, leftward and superiorly as does the remainder of the loop (Fig. 2-49). Since the initial QRS vector projects on the positive side of the X and Z lead axes, a small upward deflection (so-called delta wave) marking the onset of the R wave is recorded in these leads. Presence of the delta wave accounts for a widening of the QRS complex (0.11 to 0.14 sec.) at the expense of the PR interval. Thus, in leads X and Z the PR interval measures only 0.10 sec. or less (Fig. 2-49).

Horizontal plane loop. The initial QRS vector is oriented to the left and posteriorly but occasionally is oriented slightly anteriorly. The QRS loop is usually inscribed in a counterclockwise direction, although a figure-of-eight pattern may be recorded occasionally. The initial portion of the QRS loop and sometimes almost the entire efferent limb displays conduction delay as indicated by close spacing between dots. The maximum QRS vector is oriented posteriorly and to the left and its magnitude is often increased.

Thus an erroneous diagnosis of left ventricular hypertrophy can be made unless one realizes the initial slowing. The T loop may be opposite to the QRS loop (Fig. 2-50).

Right sagittal plane loop. The loop configuration and inscription is quite variable. When the loop is oriented inferiorly it has a clockwise direction of inscription, and when the loop is oriented superiorly it is usually inscribed in a counterclockwise direction (Fig. 2-51).

Frontal plane loop. The initial portion and the body of the QRS loop are usually oriented to the left and either superiorly or inferiorly. The direction of inscription is variable and a figure-of-eight pattern is fairly common (Fig. 2-52).

Standard 12 lead electrocardiogram. The QRS vectors oriented posteriorly, to the left and superiorly, project on the negative side of the axis of the right precordial leads, and most of the limb leads giving rise to QS complexes or predominantly negative QRS complexes, with the delta wave on the descending limb in leads V1, L2, L3, aVR, and aVF. The left precordial leads register the type of QRS complexes described for type A. The PR interval is 0.10 second or less (Fig. 2-53).

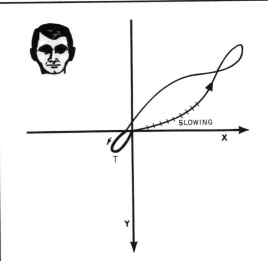

Fig. 2-52. Diagram of the frontal plane VCG in type B WPWS.

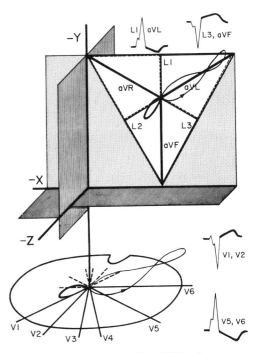

Fig. 2-53. Diagram of the 12 lead system electrocardiograms in type B WPWS.

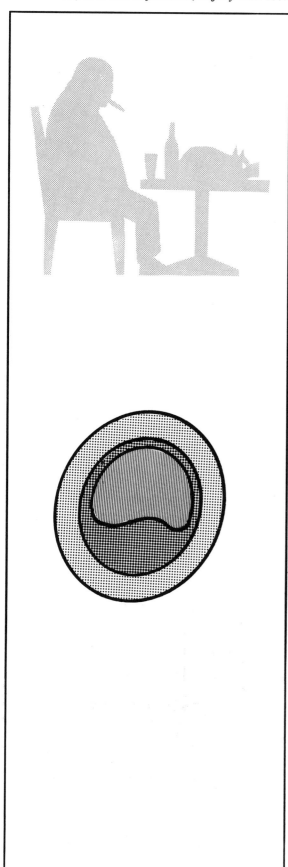

Myocardial Infarction, Injury and Ischemia

VCG IN MYOCARDIAL INFARCTION (GENERAL CONSIDERATIONS)

Pathogenesis of Myocardial Infarction

Myocardial infarction is due to a sudden, very severe diminution or interruption of blood flow to an area of the myocardium leading to its necrosis. In most cases (about 80%) a fresh coronary occlusion is present as a result of thrombosis in a sclerotic coronary artery. In other cases, occlusion may result from sloughing of atheromatous debris into the lumen of a coronary artery, intimal swelling and/or hemorrhage into an atheromatous plaque, coronary artery embolism in subacute bacterial endocarditis, syphilitic aortitis with narrowing of the coronary ostia or inflammation of the coronary arteries (thromboangitis obliterans, periarteritis nodosa, etc.).

The victim is usually a middle-aged man, of a mesomorphic build, a heavy smoker with a family history of cardiovascular disease or diabetes. Provided the attack does not cause sudden death, the patient is seized by a retrosternal pain similar to that in angina but differing in its greater, often agonizing, severity, its persistence for several hours or longer, and its failure to be relieved by nitro-glycerine. It is, moreover, accompanied, to a greater or lesser degree, by circulating collapse — pallor, sweating, dizziness and occasionally vomiting and syncope. In most cases (about 95%) there is a rise in the serum glutamic-oxalacetic transaminase (GOT); a peak level of GOT usually 2 to 10 times the normal value is reached within 48 hours. A rise in serum lactic dehydrogenase is also of diagnostic value. The vectorcardiogram or electrocardiogram usually reveals the diagnostic changes of infarction. However, a diagnosis of myocardial infarction, based on clinical evidence, should never be discounted on the basis of a normal vectorcardiogram or electrocardiogram.

Typical VCG Changes in Myocardial Infarction

From the physiologic and vectorcardiographic points of view, the infarcted area may be divided into the dead zone, the zone of injury and the zone of ischemia (Fig. 2-54).

The dead zone constitutes the central area of the infarcted region. It is composed of dead muscle fibers which are electrically inactive. This zone accounts for the changes in the initial QRS vector which points away from the site of infarction (see page 86). In vectorcardiographic loops, these changes are manifested by the 0.03 sec. QRS vector shifted in the direction opposite the site of infarction, while in scalar tracings these changes are manifested by a deep and wide Q wave in those leads which normally show very small or no q wave (Fig. 2-55).

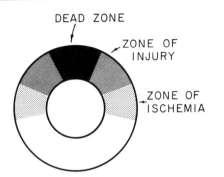

Fig. 2-54. Diagram showing the 3 zones of an infarct.

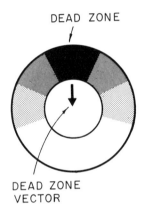

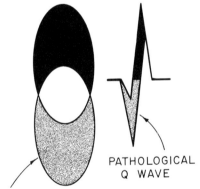

Fig. 2-55. Diagram showing the dead zone vector and how it affects the VCG loop and the scalar tracing. Shadowed area indicates a shifted portion and the black area the lost portion of the loop or scalar tracing.

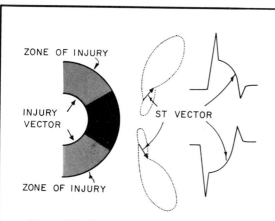

Fig. 2-56. *Diagram showing the injury zone vector and how it affects the VCG loop and the scalar tracing.*

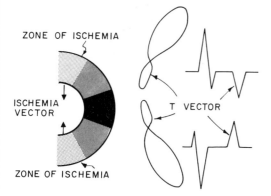

Fig. 2-57. *Diagram showing the ischemia zone vector and how it affects the VCG loop and the scalar tracing.*

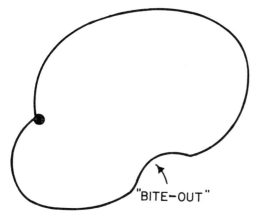

Fig. 2-58. *Diagram illustrating "bite-outs" in the QRS loop.*

The zone of injury constitutes a shell of cardiac muscle that surrounds the dead zone. It is composed of muscle fibers which do not regain a complete state of polarization with each cardiac cycle. This zone accounts for the injury vector which points toward the site of infarction (see page 86). In vectorcardiographic loops the injury vector is manifested by the ST vector whose magnitude is increased, and whose orientation points toward the location of injury, while in scalar tracings this vector is manifested by a strongly marked elevation or depression of the ST segment (Fig. 2-56).

The zone of ischemia constitutes a shell of cardiac muscle that surrounds the zone of injury. It is composed of muscle fibers that are slightly deprived of coronary blood flow. This zone accounts for the changes in the T vector, which points away from the site of infarction (see page 87). In vectorcardiographic loops these changes are manifested by a wide QRS-T angle and a more symmetrical, rounded T loop with a constant speed of inscription, while in scalar tracings these changes are manifested by an inverted (negative) T wave in leads which normally record an upright T wave (Fig. 2-57).

There are other conditions which may produce one or another of these abnormalities, but only infarction can produce all three. However, all three are present only in the acute stage of infarction. This means that the diagnosis of infarction is almost certain in the presence of all three vector abnormalities. The presence of the injury and/or ischemia vector without signs of necrosis may occur in pericarditis, chronic coronary insufficiency (angina pectoris) and some other conditions (see page 131). The presence of the infarction-like changes of the initial QRS vector with or without T vector changes sometimes may be encountered in septal hypertrophy, myocardial fibrosis, myocardial clefts, abnormal conduction and emphysema.

On the other hand, the infarction pattern in the vectorcardiogram can be masked by preexisting abnormalities (bundle branch block, hypertrophy), or by complications arising along with an infarct (bundle branch block, pericarditis). In such cases, especially in the presence of left bundle branch block, affecting the initial QRS vectors, the diagnosis of an infarction is very difficult.

Finally, it should be pointed out that in rare cases of myocardial infarction, especially when it is small or confined to the interior of the myocardium, the vectorcardiogram may be normal. It also has been found that the vectorcardiographic diagnosis of myocardial infarction in diabetic patients is more difficult. This may be explained by the fact that in patients with diabetes mellitus there occurs multifocal fibrosis of the myocardium without large unifocal infarcts. Such multifocal lesions may fail to produce typical VCG changes, but they can produce small "bite outs" occurring in the mid or terminal portions of the loop (Fig. 2-58). When their duration is more than 5 msec. and their magnitude is more than 0.10 mv they are regarded as suspicious of infarction.

VCG Course of Infarction

The vectorcardiogram is often very helpful in diagnosing the duration and timing of a myocardial infarct. The age of an infarct can be determined from the fact that the injury vector is present only during the acute stage, and that the T vector changes are present only during the recent stage.

When the vectorcardiogram displays the injury vector with or without QRS vector changes and/or T vector changes, the diagnosis of an "acute myocardial infarction" is justified (Fig. 2-59). The length of the acute stage varies from case to case and may be from a few days up to weeks. Persistence of the VCG pattern of an acute infarction for longer than this should arouse suspicion of a cardiac aneurysm.

When the injury vector has vanished and the vectorcardiogram pattern consists of the changes in the initial QRS vector and the T vector, the diagnosis of a "recent myocardial infarction" is justified (Fig. 2-60). The length of the recent stage varies from case to case and may be from a few weeks up to months or years.

At still a later period when both the injury vector and also the T vector changes have vanished, and only the changes in the initial QRS vectors remain, the diagnosis of an "old myocardial infarction" is justified (Fig. 2-61). These changes usually persist as a sign of residual fibrosis. They may diminish in size over the years as a result of shrinkage of the infarction scar and compensation by the surrounding muscle; however, only in exceptional cases is there complete normalization of the initial QRS vectors.

The evolution of an infarct can stop at the recent stage and never proceed to the chronic stage. Thus it is impossible to be sure about the age of an infarct without serial vectorcardiograms and/or the clinical history of the patient.

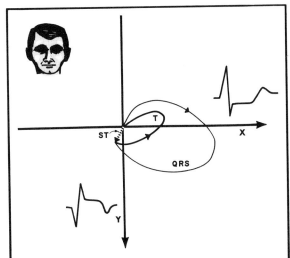

Fig. 2-59. Diagram depicting the VCG pattern of an acute myocardial infarction.

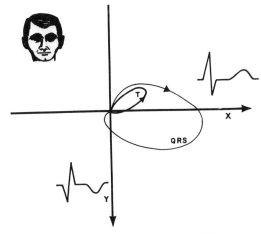

Fig. 2-60. Diagram depicting the VCG pattern of a recent myocardial infarction.

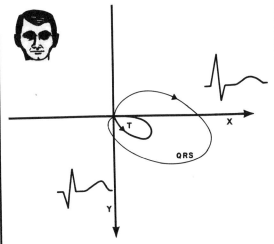

Fig. 2-61. Diagram depicting the VCG pattern of an old myocardial infarction.

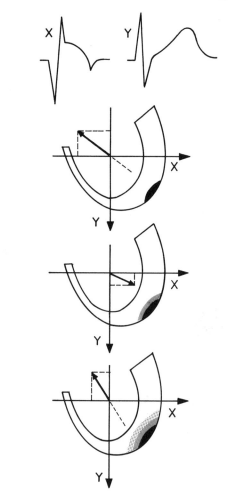

Fig. 2-62. *Diagram to illustrate the manner in which the dead zone vector, the injury vector and the T vector can be used to predict the location of an infarct.*

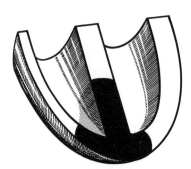

Fig. 2-63. *Diagram showing the anatomical location of an anterior infarct.*

Sites of Infarction

Myocardial infarcts are located almost exclusively in the musculature of the left ventricle. They may occur very rarely in the right ventricle and the atria, but these sites hardly ever produce recognizable VCG changes.

On the basis of the VCG pattern of myocardial infarction, an attempt can be made to localize the infarct. This is usually done by fixing the dead zone vector which points from the center of the infarct toward the center of the left ventricle. In addition, during an acute stage of infarct an attempt can be made to fix the injury vector, which has the direction of a line drawn from a center of the left ventricle toward the center of the injured region. In a similar way during a recent stage of infarction, an attempt can be made to fix the T vector which points away from the infarcted area (Fig. 2-62). If the localization by two or three of these vectors implicates distinctly different regions, one may consider more than one diagnosis.

The location of an infarct predicted from the vectorcardiogram, though often approximately correct, in many cases may be false. The main reason for getting a false location is the presence of additional factors (e.g., coexisting abnormalities of ventricular conduction), which may modify the direction of the unbalanced forces produced by an infarction.

Since anatomical localization of an infarction from the vectorcardiogram cannot be entirely correct in every individual case, and since the information regarding the anatomic site of an infarction is of doubtful clinical value (at least for the time being), pinpointed localization seems to be unrealistic. It appears that vectorcardiographically one can distinguish only four basic types of myocardial infarction:

1. Anterior infarcts
2. Lateral infarcts
3. Posterodiaphragmatic infarct
4. True posterior infarcts.

Anterior infarcts are situated in the anterior wall of the left ventricle and usually involve also the anterior part of the ventricular septum (Fig. 2-63).

Lateral infarcts involve the lateral wall of the left ventricle and may extend to the anterior wall (Fig. 2-64).

Posterodiaphragmatic infarcts are situated in the lower portion of the posterior wall of the left ventricle which, for the most part, rests on the diaphragm (Fig. 2-65).

True posterior infarcts involve some region of the posterobasal left ventricle wall (Fig. 2-66).

Another classification of infarcts is based on the extent to which the necrosis has progressed (Fig. 2-67). An infarct may be subendocardial, subepicardial, intramural (confined to the interior of the myocardium), or transmural (involving the full thickness of the myocardium). Usually an intramural infarct which does not involve the endocardium or epicardium is vectorcardiographically or electrocardiographically silent.

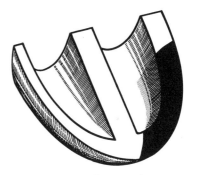

Fig. 2-64. Diagram showing the anatomical location of a lateral infarct.

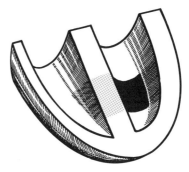

Fig. 2-65. Diagram showing the anatomical location of a postero-diaphragmatic infarct.

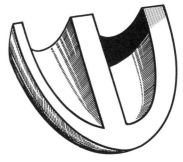

Fig. 2-66. Diagram showing the anatomical location of a true posterior infarct.

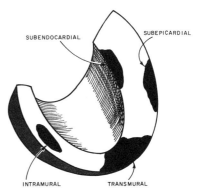

SUBENDOCARDIAL   SUBEPICARDIAL

INTRAMURAL   TRANSMURAL

Fig. 2-67. Diagram showing different locations of an infarct in relation to the thickness of the ventricular wall.

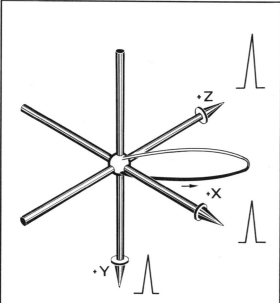

Fig. 2-68. Diagram showing the spatial QRS loop and its projections recorded in X, Y, and Z leads in anterior myocardial infarction.

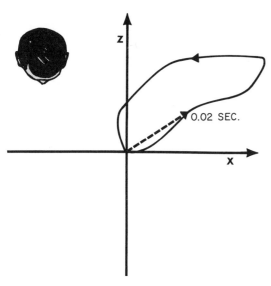

Fig. 2-69. Diagram of the horizontal plane VCG in anterior myocardial infarction.

VCG IN ANTERIOR MYOCARDIAL INFARCTION

Scalar X, Y, Z Components

The principal alteration in the spatial QRS loop is the posterior and leftward displacement of the initial vectors. This is manifested by the absence of the q wave or the presence of a very small q wave (amplitude < 0.1 mv) in lead Z. Consequently the Q/R amplitude ratio in lead Z is less than 0.1 (Fig. 2-68). The morphology of the ST and T vectors varies with the age of the infarction (see page 117).

Vectorcardiographic Loops

Characteristic findings of anterior myocardial infarction (i.e., the posterior displacement of the initial QRS vectors) are seen in the horizontal and sagittal planes which involve the Z (anterior-posterior) lead.

Horizontal plane QRS loop. The initial 0.02 sec. vector points posteriorly and to the left (i.e., it lies in the posterior left quadrant). In other words, the first 0.02 sec. of the horizontal plane loop is inscribed superiorly to the 0°-180° axis passing through the E point. When the 0.01 sec. vector points anteriorly but the 0.02 sec. vector points posteriorly, the probability of an anterior infarction remains high but is considerably reduced in the presence of left ventricular hypertrophy, especially if congestive heart failure is present.

The early portion of the efferent limb displays concavity as opposed to the normal convexity. The direction of inscription is counterclockwise; however, in some instances the initial portion may be inscribed clockwise (Fig. 2-69).

Right sagittal plane QRS loop. The initial 0.002 sec. vector is oriented posteriorly. The early portion of the efferent limb displays concavity as opposed to the normal convexity. The direction of inscription is usually clockwise (Fig. 2-70). However, if the initial portion moves posteriorly and superiorly a figure-of-eight may appear with the early portion inscribed counterclockwise, or the whole loop may be inscribed counterclockwise. The counterclockwise inscription in the presence of anterior infarction is believed to result from an associated inferior infarction.

Standard 12 Lead Electrocardiogram

The posteriorly displaced initial QRS vectors project on the negative side of the right and/or midprecordial leads axis. Consequently QS or QR patterns are recorded in leads V1-V3 or V3-V4 or V4-V5, or there is a decrease in the amplitude of the initial R wave on going from lead V1 to V4 (Fig. 2-71).

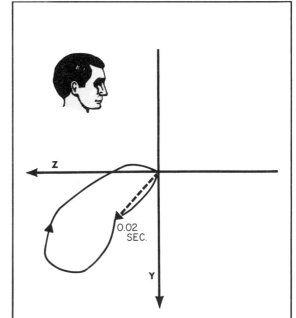

Fig. 2-70. Diagram of the right sagittal plane VCG in anterior myocardial infarction.

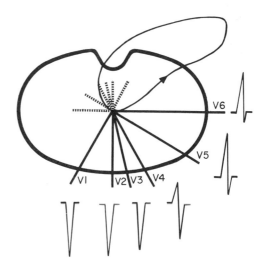

Fig. 2-71. Diagram showing the horizontal plane electrocardiograms in anterior myocardial infarction.

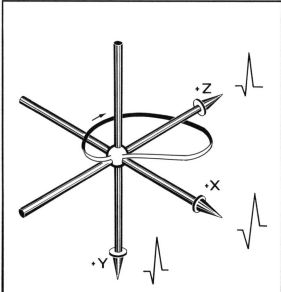

Fig. 2-72. *Diagram showing the spatial QRS loop and its projections recorded in X, Y, and Z leads in lateral myocardial infarction.*

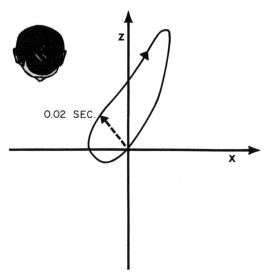

Fig. 2-73. *Diagram of the horizontal plane VCG in lateral myocardial infarction.*

VCG IN LATERAL MYOCARDIAL INFARCTION

Scalar X, Y, Z Components

The principal alteration in the spatial QRS loop is the rightward displacement of the initial vectors. This is manifested by a QR pattern with an abnormal Q wave (duration > 0.03 sec. and/or amplitude > 0.025 mv) in lead X. Consequently the Q/R amplitude ratio in this lead is greater than 0.21 (Fig. 2-72). The morphology of the ST and T vectors varies with the age of the infarction (see page 117).

Vectorcardiographic Loops

Characteristic findings of lateral myocardial infarction (i.e., the rightward displacement of the initial QRS vectors) are seen in the horizontal and frontal planes which involve the X (left to right) lead.

Horizontal plane QRS loop. The initial 0.02 sec. vector is oriented to the right and either anteriorly or posteriorly.

The initial part of the QRS loop is usually inscribed clockwise, but the remainder of the loop may be inscribed either clockwise or counterclockwise (Fig. 2-73). In the latter case the loop displays a figure-of-eight pattern. Occasionally the QRS loop may be inscribed in a normal counterclockwise direction.

Frontal plane QRS loop. The initial 0.02 sec. vector is oriented rightward and inferiorly. The direction of inscription is usually counterclockwise. The maximum QRS vector tends to assume a vertical position (Fig. 2-74).

Standard 12 Lead Electrocardiogram
The initial QRS vectors that are displaced to the right in lateral infarction, project on the negative side of the axis of leads L1 and aVL, giving rise to an abnormal Q wave in these leads (Fig. 2-75).

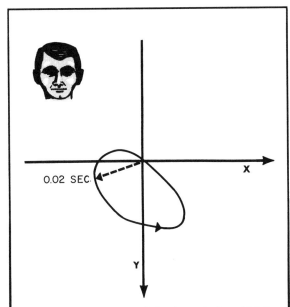

Fig. 2-74. Diagram of the frontal plane VCG in lateral myocardial infarction.

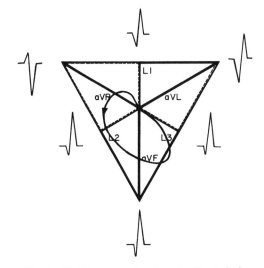

Fig. 2-75. Diagram showing the frontal plane electrocardiograms in lateral myocardial infarction.

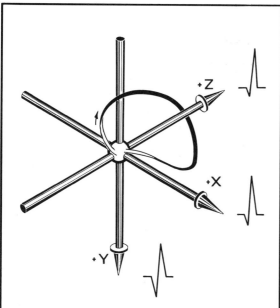

Fig. 2-76. Diagram showing the spatial QRS loop and its projections recorded in X, Y, and Z leads in postero-diaphragmatic infarct.

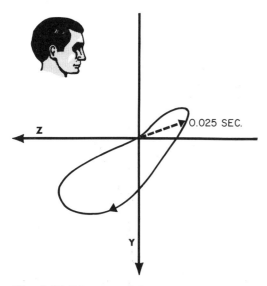

Fig. 2-77. Diagram of the right sagittal plane VCG in postero-diaphragmatic infarct.

VCG IN INFEROPOSTERIOR MYOCARDIAL INFARCTION

Scalar X, Y, Z Components

The principal alteration in the spatial QRS loop is the superior displacement of the initial vectors. This change is manifested by a pathological Q wave (duration > 0.03 sec. and/or amplitude > 0.3 mv) in lead Y. Consequently the Q/R amplitude ratio in this lead is greater than 0.22 (Fig. 2-76). Occasionally a QS complex appears in lead Y, indicating that all the QRS vectors point superiorly. The morphology of the ST and T vectors varies with the age of the infarction.

Vectorcardiographic Loops

Characteristic findings of inferior myocardial infarction (i.e., the superior displacement of the initial QRS vectors) are seen in the sagittal and frontal planes which involve the Y (superior-inferior) lead. The horizontal plane QRS remains usually normal.

Right sagittal plane QRS loop. The 0.025 second vector points superiorly and anteriorly (i.e., it lies in the anterior superior quadrant). In other words, the first 0.025 sec. of the right sagittal plane loop is inscribed superiorly to the

0°-180° axis, passing through the E point. The direction of inscription is usually normal (i.e., clockwise), although in some cases it may be partially counterclockwise (figure-of-eight pattern with a distal portion inscribed counterclockwise) or completely counterclockwise (Fig. 2-77). The counterclockwise inscription is believed to be associated with an anterior wall infarction as the initial QRS vectors point superiorly and posteriorly. The maximum QRS vector tends to be oriented more posteriorly and less inferiorly as compared with normal cases.

Frontal plane QRS loop. The initial 0.025 second vector points superiorly and either to the left or right. In other words, the first 0.025 sec. of the frontal plane loop is inscribed superiorly to the 0°-180° axis passing through the E point. The direction of inscription is almost always clockwise. Occasionally the afferent limb may return counterclockwise (figure-of-eight pattern). The maximum QRS vector usually is directed superiorly to 20° (Fig. 2-78).

Standard 12 Lead Electrocardiogram

The initial QRS vectors that are displaced superiorly in inferior infarction, project on the negative side of the L2, L3 and aVF lead axes giving rise to a pathological Q wave in these leads (Fig. 2-79).

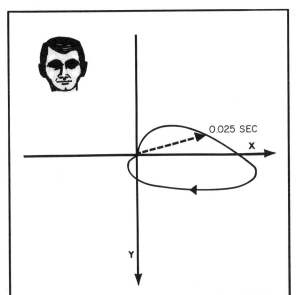

Fig. 2-78. *Diagram of the frontal plane VCG in postero-diaphragmatic infarct.*

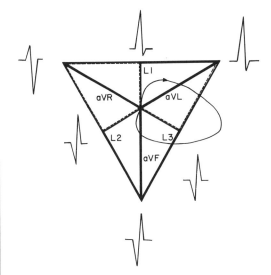

Fig. 2-79. *Diagram showing the frontal plane electrocardiograms in postero-diaphragmatic infarct.*

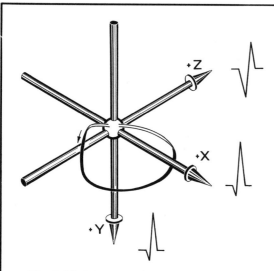

Fig. 2-80. *Diagram showing the spatial QRS loop and its projections recorded in X, Y, and Z leads in true posterior infarct.*

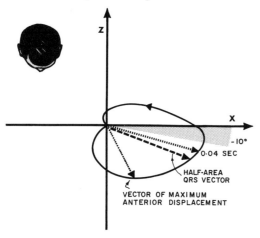

Fig. 2-81. *Diagram of the horizontal plane VCG in true posterior myocardial infarction.*

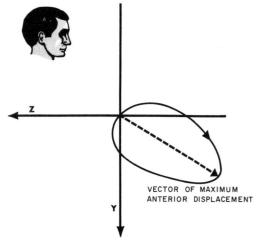

Fig. 2-82. *Diagram of the right sagittal plane VCG in true posterior myocardial infarction.*

VCG IN STRICTLY POSTERIOR MYOCARDIAL INFARCTION

Scalar X, Y, Z Components

The principal alteration in the spatial QRS loop is the anterior displacement of the initial vectors. This is manifested by a pathological Q wave (duration > 0.048 sec. and/or amplitude > 0.93 mv) in lead Z. Consequently the Q/R amplitude ratio in this lead is greater than 1.2 (Fig. 2-80). The morphology of the ST and T vectors varies with the age of the infarction (see page 117).

Vectorcardiographic Loops

Characteristic findings of strictly posterior myocardial infarction (i.e., the anterior displacement of the initial QRS vectors) are seen in the horizontal and sagittal planes which involve the Z (anterior-posterior) lead.

Horizontal plane QRS loop. More than 50 percent of the loop lies below the horizontal (i.e., the 0°-180°) axis, passing through the E point. This displacement also can be measured by the orientation of the half area or the 0.04 sec. QRS vectors, which are oriented anteriorly to 10°. The vector of maximum anterior displacement may be greater than 0.6 mv. The direction of inscription is usually counterclockwise (Fig. 2-81). Occasionally the loop may be inscribed clockwise and in such cases the differentiation from right ventricular hypertrophy is very difficult.

Right sagittal plane QRS loop. The loop is displaced anteriorly and the magnitude of the vector of maximum anterior displacement is increased. The loop inscription is usually clockwise but occasionally may be counterclockwise (Fig. 2-82).

Standard 12 Lead Electrocardiogram

The initial QRS vectors that are displaced anteriorly in strictly posterior infarction, project on the positive side of the axis of the right precordial leads. Consequently the R wave in lead V1 and/or V2 has increased amplitude and the R/S amplitude ratio in these leads often becomes equal to or greater than 1 (Fig. 2-83).

VCG IN PERI-INFARCTION BLOCK

Occurrence and the Vectorcardiographic Pattern

When the abnormal QRS vectors diagnostic of myocardial infarction are accompanied by slowly inscribed terminal vectors, which are directed in an opposite direction to that of the initial QRS vectors, such a pattern is called a peri-infarction block; and it is believed to result from a block of the inferior or superior branch of the left bundle at the periphery of the necrotic zone of the myocardium.

The overwhelming majority of cases of peri-infarction block may be divided into 2 types:

1. Peri-infarction block with the terminal QRS vectors directed to the left and superiorly, which is usually associated with anterior infarction interrupting the superior branch of the left bundle (Fig. 2-84).

2. Peri-infarction block with the terminal QRS vectors directed to the right and inferiorly, which is usually associated with inferior infarction interrupting the inferior branch of the left bundle (Fig. 2-85).

In either type of peri-infarction block the frontal plane vectorcardiogram shows a wide angle, greater than 90°, between the initial and terminal QRS vectors. Usually there is little or no prolongation of the QRS loop duration.

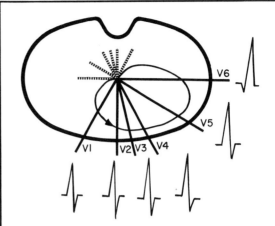

Fig. 2-83. Diagram depicting the horizontal plane electrocardiograms in true posterior myocardial infarction.

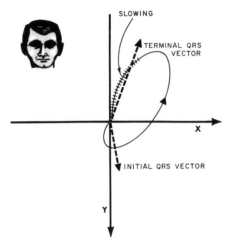

Fig. 2-84. Diagram illustrating the VCG pattern of a peri-infarction block associated with anterior infarction (as seen in the frontal plane).

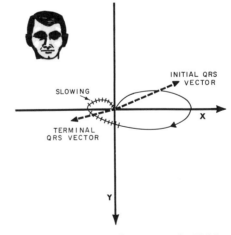

Fig. 2-85. Diagram illustrating the VCG pattern of a peri-infarction block associated with inferior infarction (as seen in the frontal plane).

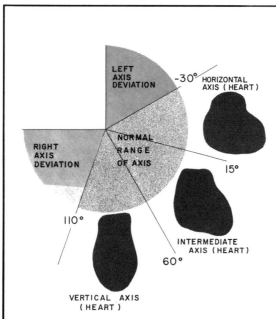

Fig. 2-86. Diagram showing the normal range of the mean electrical axis and its right and left deviation (in the frontal plane).

Miscellaneous VCG Patterns

LEFT AXIS DEVIATION

Clinical Significance

The term mean electrical axis of the heart has been adopted for the direction of the mean QRS vector in the frontal plane. Since calculation of the mean QRS vector is time-consuming, it is much more practical to use the maximum QRS vector in the frontal plane for the mean electrical axis determination (see page 61). Normally the mean electrical axis of the heart is located in the left inferior quadrant of the frontal plane (i.e., between 0° and 90°), and is influenced by the anatomical position of the heart in the chest; thus the more horizontal (or vertical) the heart position, the more horizontal (or vertical) the mean electrical axis (Fig. 2-86). However, a deviation of the axis to the right (> 90°) or to the left (< 0°) is not related to the position of the heart in the chest but is due to pathological conditions. Right axis deviation is usually due to right bundle branch block or right ventricular hypertrophy (see page 97).

Left axis deviation is one of the commonest abnormalities encountered in clinical vectorcardiography. With rare exceptions, such as, for example, left axis deviation produced by the upward displacement of the diaphragm (pregnancy, ascites, abdominal tumor), the presence of marked left axis deviation is an indication of cardiac abnormality.

Left axis deviation can be produced by several pathological conditions, the most important of which include: left bundle branch block, diffuse myocardial fibrosis secondary to coronary artery disease, or to other conditions such as cardiomyopathies, myocardial infarction, left ventricular hypertrophy, emphysema, scleroderma, cardiac amyloidosis, progressive muscular dystrophy, myocarditis, alcoholic cardiomyopathy, hyperkalemia, some congenital heart diseases (intraventricular septal defect, tricuspid atresia) and surgical injury to the superior division of the left bundle branch after heart surgery.

It is believed that left axis deviation due to conditions other than myocardial infarction results from involvement of the anterior superior fibers of the left bundle by fibrosis or other lesion. As a consequence of this, depolarization of the left ventricle proceeds by way of the posterior-inferior fibers, causing the mean electrical axis to be oriented superiorly and to the left.

Vectorcardiographic Pattern

Left axis deviation is characterized by a superior and leftward displacement of the QRS loop in the frontal plane. Consequently the 0.025 sec. vector and/or maximum QRS vector is located superiorly to the 0°-180° axis. However, a mild left axis deviation may be considered even if the mean or maximum QRS vector lies between +10° and 0°. The entire QRS loop or a significant portion of its efferent limb is inscribed in a clockwise direction (Fig. 2-87).

In the right sagittal plane the QRS loop shows a posterior-superior displacement of the body and/or terminal vectors (Fig. 2-88).

Predominantly superior orientation of QRS vectors is manifested by a deep S wave (which is greater than R wave in lead Y.

The 12 Lead ECG

Left axis deviation is characterized by a large S wave in leads L3 and aVF and by a large R wave in L1, which is greater than R wave in L2 and L3 (Fig. 2-89).

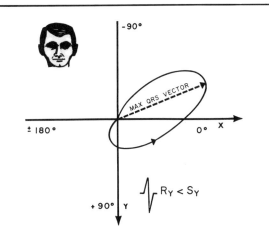

Fig. 2-87. Diagram of the frontal plane QRS loop in left axis deviation.

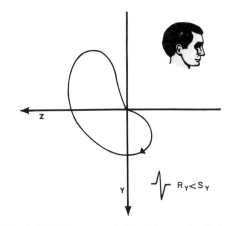

Fig. 2-88. Diagram of the right sagittal plane QRS loop in left axis deviation.

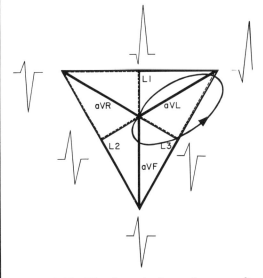

Fig. 2-89. The frontal plane electrocardiograms in left axis deviation.

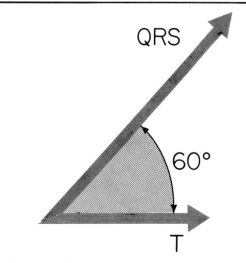

Fig. 2-90. Diagram showing the normal range of the QRS-T angle (in the horizontal plane).

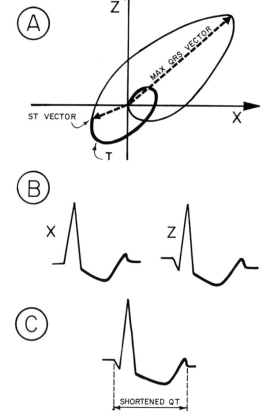

Fig. 2-91. Diagram illustrating the VCG and ECG changes due to digitalis: A. ST vector and small T loop; B. ST segment of sagging configuration and small T wave; C. shortening of the Q-T interval.

NONSPECIFIC ST-T VECTOR CHANGES

Definition and Occurrence

In normal adults the orientation of the T vectors and QRS vectors is relatively parallel, so that the QRS-T angle in the horizontal plane is less than 60° (Fig. 2-90). Only in the very young and in the elderly this angle may be wide (90° or more). An angular divergence of the maximum QRS vector and the maximum T vector greater than 60° is regarded as a T vector abnormality.

From a basic vectorcardiographic standpoint, all T vector abnormalities may be divided into two types. The first, called a primary T vector abnormality, is due to alterations in the state of cardiac muscle that affect the repolarization process. The second type, called a secondary T vector abnormality, depends upon changes in the depolarization process. Secondary T vector abnormalities occur, for example, in ventricular conduction disturbances or ventricular hypertrophy. Secondary T vector abnormalities are associated with an unchanged ventricular gradient (see page 27).

Primary T vector abnormalities are associated with a changed ventricular gradient. They may occur in a host of different conditions, both normal and abnormal, and therefore they are also called nonspecific changes. Usually, primary T vector changes result from local regions of ischemia, ventricular hypertrophy, the use of digitalis or other drugs (atropine, tricyclic anti-depressants), myocarditis, pericarditis, alcoholic cardiomyopathy, severe infections of any sort, metabolic and endocrine disturbances (e.g., acidosis, hypothyroidism), hypopotassemia, hyperpotassemia, intracranial injury, the smoking of tobacco, and some physiological conditions (pregnancy, adolescence, drinking of iced water, belonging to the black race). In fact any factor which can alter biochemical structure of the heart fiber may alter the order of repolarization process and lead to T vector abnormalities. Thus it is obvious that on vectorcardiographic grounds one can describe such abnormalities only as "nonspecific primary T vector (or wave) changes." Any etiological factor can be suggested only by examination of the associated clinical picture.

Digitalis Effect

Primary T vector changes produced by digitalis are associated with characteristic ST vector changes and may be reported as "primary ST-T change, probably due to digitalis" or "probably digitalis effect."

In a vectorcardiographic loop there is present an ST vector pointing in an opposite direction to that of the maximum QRS vector. In addition, the T loop is small but normally oriented (Fig. 2-91A). In leads X, Y, standard limb leads and the left precordial leads, the ST segment assumes a sagging configuration. The T wave is low giving the appearance of a (−+) biphasic T wave or is included as an inverted T wave in the depressed ST segment. In addition, there is a shortening of the Q-T interval (Fig. 2-91B, C). These findings result from an adequate digitalization. Over-digitalization usually leads to various arrhythmias (bradycardia, AV block, ventricular premature contractions).

Ischemic Pattern

It is believed that primary T vector changes due to local ischemia usually show characteristic changes. In such cases there is some justification for making a more specific interpretation, namely "primary T (or ST-T) vector changes probably due to ischemia."

The ischemic T loop is usually more symmetrical, (i.e., the efferent and afferent limbs are of equal length), rounded and inscribed with a constant speed, thus giving the appearance of a dense loop with closely spaced timing dots. The maximum T vector usually points anteriorly and slightly rightward (i.e., away from the general location of the left ventricle in the chest which is much more often affected by the ischemia than the right ventricle). The ST vector is often present and its orientation may be either opposite or parallel to that of the maximum T vector (Fig. 2-92A).

Scalar tracings (X, Y, standard limb leads, and the left precordial leads) display inverted T waves; however, they also may be flat or diphasic. The inverted T wave has symmetrical configuration (i.e., its downstroke and upstroke have similar slopes in relation to the vertical line). In addition, the T wave is peaked (Fig. 2-92B). The ST segment may be isoelectric, elevated (0.1 mv or more) or depressed (0.05 mv or less).

The above described ST-T vector abnormalities also may be found in many other conditions. Therefore, one should be cautious in making the diagnosis of ischemia from a given ST-T vector abnormality, unless there is other clinical evidence in favor of such a diagnosis.

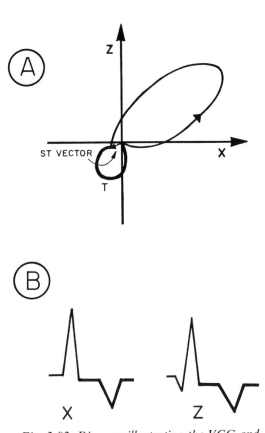

Fig. 2-92. Diagram illustrating the VCG and ECG changes due to ischemia: A. Rounded T loop and small ST vector; B. Symmetrical T wave and elevated or depressed ST segment.

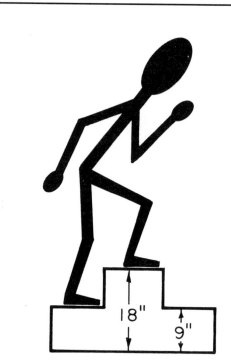

Fig. 2-93. Diagram illustrating the Master "2-step" test.

ANGINA PECTORIS

Origin and Occurrence

Angina pectoris is characterized by a sudden, severe retrosternal pain, which usually is precipitated by an exertion, overeating or excitement, and is relieved quickly by rest and nitroglycerin.

Angina pectoris results from an acute inadequacy of coronary blood flow which leads only to myocardial hypoxia, but is not severe enough to cause necrosis (infarction). It is usually associated with arteriosclerosis of the coronary arteries which may be further narrowed by spasm, edema or subintimal hemorrhage within an atherosclerotic plaque. However, there are many other pathologic conditions which can induce myocardial hypoxia. These conditions include left ventricular hypertrophy, aortic stenosis, pulmonary hypertension, polycythemia, Buerger's disease, rheumatic fever, and anemia.

In cases of "pure angina pectoris," that is angina without evidence of previous or present infarction, cardiac enlargement or myocardial failure, the vectorcardiogram may show signs of ischemia and sometimes also injury (see page 114) but usually is within normal limits. Therefore a diagnosis of pure angina pectoris may be made in the absence of an abnormal vectorcardiogram. On the other hand, an abnormal vectorcardiogram does not necessarily represent an evidence of angina pectoris. Because the diagnosis of this condition carries such serious import to patients, it should be made only when a characteristic history is given.

The Exercise Test

Indications. In cases where the diagnosis of angina pectoris on clinical grounds is uncertain, or the resting vectorcardiogram shows no diagnostically significant changes, the exercise test may be of some help, provided it is performed properly and interpreted with discretion. This is based on the assumption that by means of exercise the demands placed on the coronary blood supply of the myocardium is increased, thus producing relative ischemia and/or injury in patients with impaired coronary blood flow due to narrowing of the coronary arteries.

The exercise test is contraindicated in patients with a suspected recent or old myocardial infarction, in patients over 70 years of age or in poor general health, in the absence of proper equipment for resuscitation and defibrilation, and in the absence of direct supervision by a physician trained in VCG interpretation and resuscitation procedures. It also should be kept in mind that in patients who have hypokalemia or have been on digitalis therapy, or their VCG demonstrates ventricular hypertrophy, the exercise test is useless.

The work load. The most widely used exercise tests are the Master Two-Step Test and walking or running on a motor-driven treadmill.

In Master's test the patient climbs up two steps (height of each step being 9 inches) and descends the steps on the other side thus completing one trip (Fig. 2-93). The total number of trips to be taken without pause in a 1½-minute interval has been standardized for the patient's sex, age and weight and listed in special tables (Table 2-1) originally reported by Master (Am. Heart J., 10:497, 1935).

Walking or running on the treadmill may be performed at a constant speed of 3-6 mph on a 10 percent grade (Fig. 2-94) or in several stages each lasting 2-3 minutes and involving a different speed and grade. In the latter case the treadmill test starts at 1-2 mph on a 0 or 2 percent grade and gradually progresses to the terminal stage with the speed of 6 mph and on a 10 percent grade. The test is terminated when the patient is unable or unwilling to continue (usually after 10-15 minutes).

The patient is instructed to report any anginal or other symptoms that may occur during the exercise test. To minimize the risk of the test, especially for higher level stress,

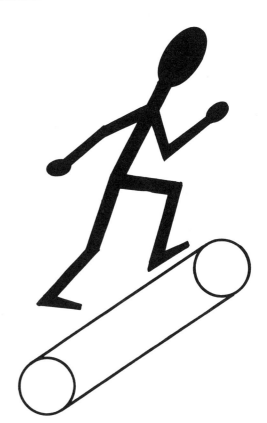

Fig. 2-94. Diagram illustrating the motor-driven treadmill.

TABLE 2-1
STANDARD NUMBER OF ASCENTS FOR MALES

Weight (lb.)	Age in Years												
	5–9	10–14	15–19	20–24	25–29	30–34	35–39	40–44	45–49	50–54	55–59	60–64	65–69
40–49	35	36											
50–59	33	35	32										
60–69	31	33	31										
70–79	28	32	30										
80–89	26	30	29	29	29	28	27	27	26	25	25	24	23
90–99	24	29	28	28	28	27	27	26	25	25	24	23	22
100–109	22	27	27	28	28	27	26	25	25	24	23	22	22
110–119	20	26	26	27	27	26	25	25	24	23	23	22	21
120–129	18	24	25	26	27	26	25	24	23	23	22	21	20
130–139	16	23	24	25	26	25	24	23	23	22	21	20	20
140–149		21	23	24	25	24	24	23	22	21	20	20	19
150–159		20	22	24	25	24	23	22	21	20	20	19	18
160–169		18	21	23	24	23	22	22	21	20	19	18	18
170–179			20	22	23	23	22	21	20	19	18	18	17
180–189			19	21	23	22	21	20	19	19	18	17	16
190–199			18	20	22	21	21	20	19	18	17	16	15
200–209				19	21	21	20	19	18	17	16	16	15
210–219				18	21	20	19	18	17	17	16	15	14
220–229				17	20	20	19	18	17	16	15	14	13

STANDARD NUMBER OF ASCENTS FOR FEMALES

Weight (lb.)	Age in Years												
	5–9	10–14	15–19	20–24	25–29	30–34	35–39	40–44	45–49	50–54	55–59	60–64	65–69
40–49	35	35	33										
50–59	33	33	32										
60–69	31	32	30										
70–79	28	30	29										
80–89	26	28	28	28	28	27	26	24	23	22	21	21	20
90–99	24	27	26	27	26	25	24	23	22	22	21	20	19
100–109	22	25	25	26	26	25	24	23	22	21	20	19	18
110–119	20	23	23	25	25	24	23	22	21	20	19	18	18
120–129	18	22	22	24	24	23	22	21	20	19	19	18	17
130–139	16	20	20	23	23	22	21	20	19	19	18	17	16
140–149		18	19	22	22	21	20	19	19	18	17	16	16
150–159		17	17	21	20	20	19	19	18	17	16	16	15
160–169		15	16	20	19	19	18	18	17	16	16	15	14
170–179		13	14	19	18	18	17	17	16	16	15	14	13
180–189			13	18	17	17	17	16	16	15	14	14	13
190–199			12	17	16	16	16	15	15	14	13	13	12
200–209				16	15	15	15	14	14	13	13	12	11
210–219				15	14	14	14	13	13	13	12	11	11
220–229				14	13	13	13	13	12	12	11	11	10

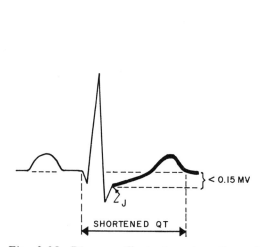

Fig. 2-95. Diagram illustrating the effect of exercise on the scalar tracing in normal subjects.

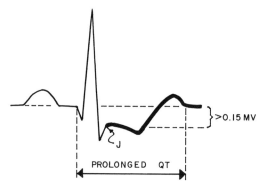

Fig. 2-96. Diagram illustrating the effect of exercise on the scalar tracing in subjects with coronary heart disease.

a constant monitoring is recommended during the test and recovery. The test is terminated when the patient complains of discomfort or pain, or an ataxic gait appears or runs of three or more ventricular premature beats develops.

Criteria for abnormality. VCG changes due to exercise can be observed in the record taken during, immediately after and 3 minutes (or 5 minutes) after the test. Virtually all the diagnostic information that can be revealed in post-exercise records can be found in leads X and Y or L1 and V5.

In a healthy subject the VCG upon exercise demonstrates an increased heart rate, a shortening of the PR interval, a shortening of the QT interval and a depression of the J point up to 0.15 mv with an upward sloping ST segment (Fig. 2-95).

In the patient with a latent or subclinical coronary heart disease upon exercise the VCG may show one or more of the following findings:

1. A depression of the J point more than 0.15 mv with a flat or downward sloping ST segment (Fig. 2-96);
2. A depression of the J point more than 0.2 mv with a flat or downward or upward sloping ST segment;
3. Abnormal widening of the QRS-T angle which produces inverted T waves in leads usually recording upright QRS complex (X, Y, L1, L2, V4-V6);
4. Increased duration of the QRS complex;
5. The occurrence of extrasystoles of ventricular origin;
6. A prolonged QT interval (Fig. 2-96).

It is believed that in about 40 to 80 percent of patients with established angina pectoris show one or more of the above changes. However, in a considerable percentage of patients, the exercise test produces false negative results. On the other hand, some normal individuals, especially those with vasoregulatory asthenia, may have pathological ST segment depression during and following exercise. Low specificity of the exercise test in diagnosis of angina pectoris also can be attributed to the following factors.

1. The work load has not been sufficiently standardized. For a high degree of standardization, work loading must be adjusted not only to constitutional variables but also to such factors as, for example, occupation and an everyday physical activity. It is obvious that young persons and those accustomed to hard physical work can perform tasks that cannot be expected of people out of training, sedentary workers, or the elderly.

2. Tachycardia and hyperventilation during and after exercise can by themselves produce significant changes of the ST and T vectors, even in normal subjects. These changes may be precipitated with particular ease in patients with LVH.

Part 3
Vectorcardiogram
Diagnostic Evaluation

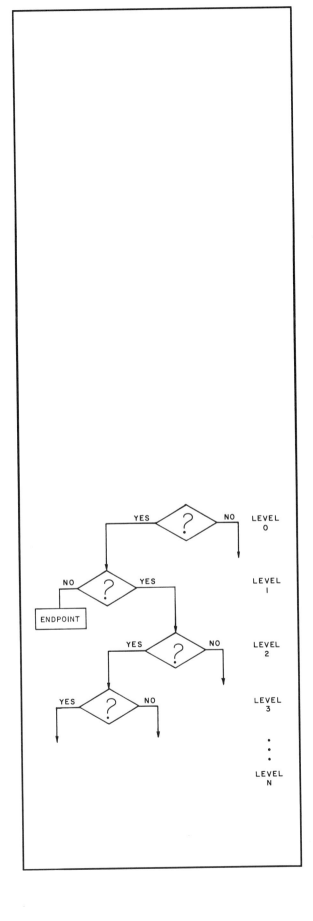

Differentiation Between Normal and Abnormal Vectorcardiograms

LOGICAL APPROACH TO DIAGNOSING VECTORCARDIOGRAMS

The Role of Logic

Logic states what follows from what, and is used as a tool of correct reasoning. It specifies rules for the testing of known conditions against established criteria, to draw conclusions and decide what action to take.

For example, before leaving the house in the morning an individual decides whether or not to wear a topcoat. He probably thinks: *If it is raining, or if rain is forecast, or if the temperature is below fifty degrees, or if I shall be coming home late, then I shall wear a topcoat.* If any one of the four conditions is satisfied, then he will wear his topcoat.

Another way of expressing the same logic is: *If it is not raining, and if rain is not forecast, and if the temperature is fifty or above, and I am coming home for dinner, then I shall not wear a topcoat.* In this case, all four conditions must be satisfied if he is not to wear his topcoat. The conditions are the reasoning or logic which lead to the conclusion or decision. Together they make up the process of making a decision.

The very same pattern of reasoning is followed by the physician who is evaluating the vectorcardiogram. For example, he may think that if the QRS duration is greater than 0.12 sec., and the horizontal plane QRS loop is inscribed clockwise, and there is a slowing of the midportion and terminal of the QRS loop, and the T loop is in the completely opposite direction to the maximal QRS vector (i.e., the QRS-T angle > 180°), then he should make the diagnosis of complete left bundle branch block.

There are two convenient methods, which may be used to formulate logic, that enter into vectorcardiographic diagnosis. One is based on decision trees and the other on decision tables. The latter method is presented on page 170.

IF CONDITIONS
① —
② —
•
•
THEN ACTION(S)
① —
•
•

IF
① QRS DURATION ⩾ 0·12 SEC.
② HORIZONTAL PLANE QRS LOOP CW
③ SLOWING OF THE MID AND TERMINAL PORTION
④ QRS-T ANGLE ⩾180 °

THEN
◯ COMPLETE LBBB PRESENT

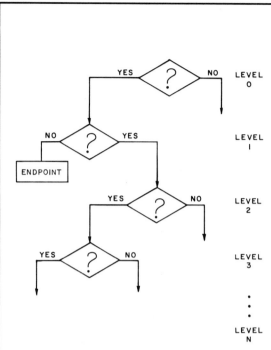

Fig. 3-1. The decision tree structure.

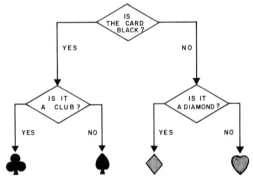

Fig. 3-2. Decision tree for determining the suit of a playing card.

Decision Tree Structure

The decision tree is a structure composed of nodes representing questions (tests) from which "yes" and "no" branches extend to other nodes. Nodes and branches are arrayed in successive levels, the highest level being the "zeroth" level, the next to the highest being the "first" level, and so forth. Unless a node is an endpoint, it is connected to two lower nodes and, through them, to any number of still lower nodes. Endpoints are nodes connected to a higher node and to no lower nodes (Fig. 3-1). Depending on the result of the test, a particular branch to a lower node is taken, and the process is repeated until an endpoint is reached. At each endpoint one of the alternatives available to a decision maker is specified. Reaching an endpoint in the tree is equivalent to taking this action.

This method is effective in reducing the number of steps needed to evaluate data. For example, to determine the suit of a playing card by this method, only two questions are to be asked (Fig. 3-2). The first question could be: Is the card black? If the answer were yes then the second question could be: Is it a club? If the answer to the first question were no then the next question could be: Is it a diamond? On this method is also based the popular game of Twenty Questions when only yes and no are allowed as answers; twenty such questions cover 1048576 alternatives. If the evaluation of VCG items were arranged to be dichotomous so that only yes and no answers were necessary, then answering only 10 questions would cover 1024 different diagnostic categories (far above the number presently distinguished by medical knowledge).

Decision Trees for Evaluation of VCG

The logic involved in diagnosing vectorcardiograms may be expressed in the form of a decision tree, shown in Figure 3-3. This tree is not unique and one could construct an entirely different tree if another sequence of tests were used. The problem, naturally, is to construct a tree with the number of tests reduced to a minimum.

The advantage of the decision tree is that it presents a step-by-step procedure for carrying out the evaluation of the vectorcardiogram, without the necessity of checking all VCG items. For example, inferior myocardial infarction may be diagnosed according to the tree from Figure 3-3 by evaluating only two VCG items, namely: initial QRS vector directed anteriorly, and initial QRS vector directed superiorly.

Although the use of the decision tree technique is very helpful in carrying out diagnostic evaluation, it is not meant to replace the physician's intuitive methods of reasoning. Rather, the decision tree technique should be considered as an aid to increasing the efficiency of the process of making a diagnostic decision by providing mechanical checks of the sequence of steps by which VCG data should be evaluated.

The use of the decision tree technique is based on the assumption that vectorcardiographic items must either be present or absent in a particular diagnostic category. In many cases, however, vectorcardiographic items are not mutually exclusive, rather, they overlap considerably. In these cases, the diagnosis must be qualified on a statistical basis.

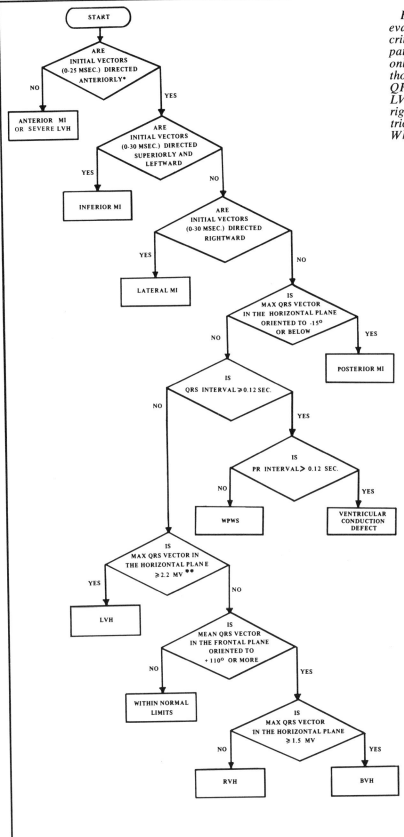

Fig. 3-3. Decision tree for the diagnostic evaluation of vectorcardiographic data. *This criterion is satisfied in about 30 percent of patients with LVH. **This criterion is valid only for patients below 50 years of age; for those above 50 the critical value of the maximal QRS vector in the HP is 1.8 mv. Abbreviations: LVH—left ventricular hypertrophy; RVH— right ventricular hypertrophy; BVH—biventricular hypertrophy; WPWS—Wolff-Parkinson-White syndrome.

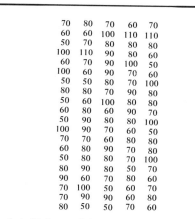

70	80	70	60	70
60	60	100	110	110
50	70	80	80	80
100	110	90	80	60
60	70	90	100	50
100	60	90	70	60
50	50	80	70	100
80	80	70	90	80
50	60	100	80	80
60	80	60	90	70
50	90	80	80	100
100	90	70	60	50
70	70	60	80	80
60	80	90	70	80
50	80	80	70	100
80	90	80	50	70
90	60	70	80	60
70	100	50	60	70
70	90	90	60	80
80	50	50	70	60

Fig. 3-4. Values of the QRS duration measured in 100 records.

50	60	70	80	90	100	110
50	60	70	80	90	100	110
50	60	70	80	90	100	110
50	60	70	80	90	100	
50	60	70	80	90	100	
50	60	70	80	90	100	
50	60	70	80	90	100	
50	60	70	80	90	100	
50	60	70	80	90	100	
50	60	70	80	90	100	
50	60	70	80	90		
50	60	70	80	90		
	60	70	80	90		
	60	70	80			
	60	70	80			
	60	70	80			
	60	70	80			
		70	80			
		70	80			
		70	80			
			80			
			80			
			80			
			80			
			80			

Fig. 3-5. Frequency distribution table for the data listed in Figure 3-4.

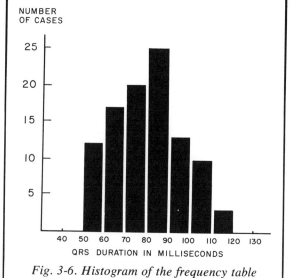

Fig. 3-6. Histogram of the frequency table from Figure 3-5.

STATISTICAL ANALYSIS OF VECTORCARDIOGRAMS

Statistical Grouping of Data

Statistics are aimed at evaluating a selected property of a mass of individual items by means of grouping the data into a number of classes and by analyzing the frequency of each class.

The simplest method of statistical grouping of data is that of the frequency distribution table, or simply the frequency table; it shows the frequencies with which a given item is distributed among the chosen classes. The construction of a frequency table is illustrated by the following example. Suppose that the QRS duration (in milliseconds) was measured in 100 records and the values were listed in the order in which they were obtained (Fig. 3-4). Because the number of observations is large and there is a considerable degree of variability of data, it is convenient to group the data into classes. This grouping requires that the range of the values be divided into equal divisions or classes. In our example, the lowest value is 50 and the highest value is 110, hence the range of values is from 50 to 110, or 60. We can choose a class width of 10 and arrange the measurements in classes of equal width with boundaries 50 and (under) 60, 60 and (under) 70 . . . 110 and (under) 120. This way all our measurements may be divided into 7 classes (Fig. 3-5). For practical consideration, the number of classes should be between 6 and 15. With fewer than 6 classes, there is insufficient detail in the table; and with more than 15 classes, excessive detail spoils the usual presentation of the data as a group.

The number of items in a class is called the frequency of that class. In general, the frequency is the number of times an item occurs. The total number of items, which is the sum of all class frequencies, is called the total frequency. The relative frequency of a class is the frequency of that class expressed as a percentage of the total frequency. For instance, in Figure 3-5 the frequency of QRS duration between 80 and 90 milliseconds is 25 and the corresponding relative frequency is 25 percent, because 25 out of 100 is 25 percent.

A graph of a frequency table is called a histogram. The histogram of the frequency table from Figure 3-5 is shown in Figure 3-6. A histogram is constructed by erecting upon the class intervals rectangles whose altitudes are equal to the frequencies. Since the bases of the rectangles are of the same length, the areas of the rectangles are proportional to the frequencies. For instance, the frequency of the QRS duration between 70 msec. and 80 msec. is twice as large as that of the QRS duration between 100 msec. and 110 msec. The areas of the two corresponding rectangles also maintain such a relation. The ratio of the area of a rectangle to the total area of all rectangles is the relative frequency of that class. For example, the area of the rectangle representing the QRS duration 100-110 msec. is 10 percent of the total area.

The most useful property of a histogram is its ability to provide the information about the position of the central value, about the degree of spread (or dispersion) around the central value, and about the degree of the lack of symmetry (or skewness).

By joining the adjacent midpoints of the upper bases of rectangles with line segments, as indicated in Figure 3-7, one obtains a frequency polygon. When the polygon is continued to the horizontal axis just outside the range of values, as in the figure, the total area under the polygon is equal to that of the histogram. The frequency polygon, with its line segments sloping upward and downward, gives a picture of the way in which frequency of occurrence varies over the complete gamut of values.

Measures of Central Tendency

Very often it becomes desirable to reduce the mass of data to a few numbers that can represent all the data and yet yield meaningful information. This can be accomplished by calculating an average which summarizes the central tendency of the data and by calculating the degree of dispersion of the data about a central value.

There are three kinds of "averages" used. The most common is the arithmetic average, or arithmetic mean, which represents the sum of the values of the observations (items) divided by the number of observations (Fig. 3-8). The arithmetic mean is usually designated by the symbol $\overline{X}$ which is read X-bar. The computation of the arithmetic mean can be described by the following expression

$$\overline{X} - \frac{\Sigma X}{N}$$

where the symbol Σ (capital sigma, the Greek letter for S) is used to represent the operation of summing. The symbol

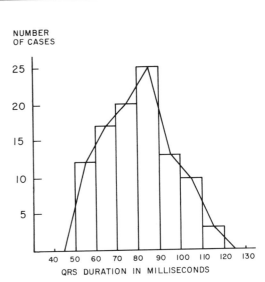

Fig. 3-7. Histogram and frequency polygon of the frequency table from Figure 3-5.

ITEM	VALUE
X_1	60
X_2	80
X_3	80
X_4	70
X_5	90
X_6	80
X_7	70
X_8	60
X_9	80
X_{10}	80
X_{11}	90
X_{12}	60
X_{13}	50
X_{14}	90
X_{15}	80
X_{16}	90
X_{17}	80
X_{18}	60
X_{19}	70
X_{20}	80

$$\text{SUM} = \sum_{i=1}^{20} X_i = 1500$$

$$\overline{X} = \frac{1500}{20} = 75$$

Fig. 3-8. Example to illustrate the calculation of the arithmetic mean.

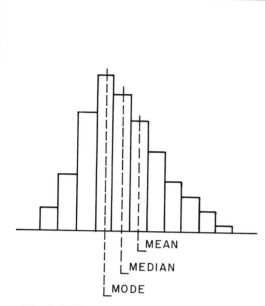

Fig. 3-9. *The mean, median and mode in a sample histogram.*

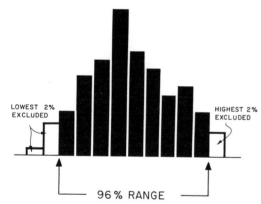

Fig. 3-10. *Diagram to illustrate the concept of the 96 percentile range.*

X represents an individual observation (item) and may be identified by a serial number: 1 for the first, 2 for the second, etc., and n for the nth. This general serial number is usually designated by the symbol i and written as a subscript (i.e., X_1 is the first observation, and X_i is the ith observation). For example, if one deals with 4 observations whose values are denoted by X_1, X_2, X_3, and X_4, the mean value is calculated according to the formula

$$\overline{X} = \frac{X_1 + X_2 + X_3 + X_4}{4}.$$

This procedure may be generalized to cover all cases. Thus, for N observations the arithmetic mean is given by the formula

$$\overline{X} = \frac{X_1 + X_2 + X_3 + \cdots + X_N}{N} \text{ or } \overline{X} = \frac{\sum_{i=1}^{N} X_i}{N}$$

where the expression $\sum_{i=1}^{N} X_i$ indicates that we are adding the Xs with subscripts from 1 to N. To illustrate the use of this formula, let us refer to Figure 3-8. It lists the measurements of the QRS duration obtained in 20 records. When all these measurements are summed up and divided by 20, we find that the mean, namely the "average" QRS duration, is 75 msec.

The median is another kind of an average. It represents the middle value (i.e., the value above which lie 50 percent of the cases and below which lie 50 percent of the cases). The mode is defined as the value which is most frequently obtained (Fig. 3-9).

Measures of Variability

The simplest measure of variability (or dispersion) is the range of data, that is, the distance between the smallest item and the largest in the distribution. Frequently the range is expressed by merely giving the smallest and the largest items. For example, in the distribution of the QRS duration given in Figure 3-4 the smallest value is 50 msec. and the largest value is 110 msec.; the range therefore is $50 - 110$ or $110 - 50 = 60$. A serious weakness of such a measure of dispersion is that it is based on only two items, and tells nothing about the manner in which the other items scatter. Furthermore, if there are one or more atypical observations (measurements) they make the range somewhat capricious.

A more accurate measure of dispersion is the 96 percentile range which is obtained as follows. The distribution ordinate is divided into 100 equal intervals. The smallest item is obtained after eliminating 2 percent of cases at the "minimal" end of the distribution, and the largest item is obtained after eliminating 2 percent of cases at the "maximal" end of the distribution (Fig. 3-10). This measure of dispersion makes use of slightly more information than does the total range, but it does not lend itself to further mathematical treatment. The 96 percent range is used only in those cases where the distribution is not symmetrical and a more accurate measure of variability cannot be computed.

A good measure of variation is found by averaging the deviations from the mean, where these deviations are taken without regard to sign. This is called the mean deviation (M.D.) and is calculated according to the formula

$$\text{M.D.} = \frac{\sum_{i=1}^{N} (X_i - \overline{X})}{N}$$

where the symbol $(X_i - \overline{X})$ represents the deviation of the ith item from the mean, and N represents the entire number of items in a sample. A simple example of the use of this formula is given in Figure 3-11. The first column represents 20 measurements of the QRS duration. The mean QRS duration is readily found to be 75 msec. The next column represents the deviations from the mean. If we change all the minus signs to plus, we find that the sum of these deviations is 220. Since there are 20 deviations, then the mean deviation is $220 \div 20 = 11$ msec. Thus the QRS durations deviate "on an average" by 11 msec. from the mean QRS duration of 75 msec.

The best and the most useful measure of dispersion is the standard deviation. In computing the standard deviation, the deviations from the mean are first squared. Next, the squared deviations are averaged by dividing their total by the number of deviations. The average of the squared deviations is called the variance. The positive square root of the variance is defined as the standard deviation. In symbols, if $(X_i - \overline{X})$ represents the deviation of the ith individual item from the mean, and $\sum_{i=1}^{N} (X_i - \overline{X})^2$ represents the sum of the squares of all the deviations, then the variance is given by the formula

$$s^2 = \frac{\sum_{i=1}^{N} (X_i - \overline{X})^2}{N}.$$

Hence, the standard deviation is given by

$$s = \sqrt{\frac{\sum_{i=1}^{N} (X_i - \overline{X})^2}{N}}.$$

The computation of the variance and standard deviation is illustrated in Figure 3-12. The mean is found to be 75 msec. The squares of the deviations appear in the second column with a sum of 2900. Therefore, the variance is 144 and the standard deviation is 12.

The standard deviation that applies to the entire population of data is denoted by the Greek letter σ (small sigma). One can estimate its value from a knowledge of the standard deviation of a sample drawn from that population.

In statistics, population refers to all the objects of a defined kind in existence in some specified universe; for example, all the adult males in the United States constitute a population, as do all the subjects suffering from myocardial infarction. In practice, it is much easier to estimate a given characteristic of a population by measuring the correspond-

QRS DURATION	DEVIATION
(X_i)	$(X_i - \overline{X})$
60	15
80	-5
80	-5
70	5
90	-15
80	-5
70	5
60	15
80	-5
80	-5
90	-15
60	15
50	25
90	-15
80	-5
90	-15
80	-5
60	15
70	5
90	-15
SUM 1510	220

$$\overline{X} = \frac{1510}{20} = 75$$

$$\text{M.D.} = \frac{220}{20} = 11$$

Fig. 3-11. Example to illustrate the calculation of the mean deviation.

QRS DURATION	SQUARED DEVIATION
(X_i)	$(X_i - \overline{X})^2$
60	225
80	25
80	25
70	25
90	225
80	25
70	25
60	225
80	25
80	25
90	225
60	225
50	625
90	225
80	25
90	225
80	25
60	225
70	25
90	225
SUM 1510	2900

$$\overline{X} = \frac{1510}{20} = 75$$

$$\text{S.D.} = \sqrt{\frac{2900}{20}} = 12$$

Fig. 3-12. Example to illustrate the calculation of the standard deviation.

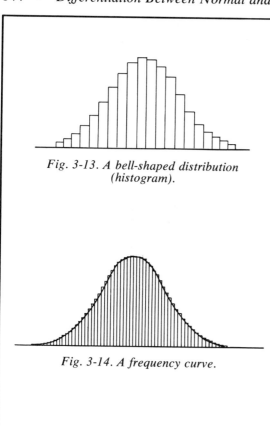

Fig. 3-13. A bell-shaped distribution (histogram).

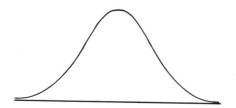

Fig. 3-14. A frequency curve.

Fig. 3-15. The normal distribution curve.

ing characteristic of a sample from the population in question.

Normal Distribution

Although frequency distribution can assume almost any shape or form, there are certain standard types which fit most distributions one meets in actual practice. Foremost among these is the aptly described bell-shaped (or normal) distribution, which is illustrated by the histogram of Figure 3-13. If the histogram of Figure 3-13 were constructed by grouping the measurements into classes of very small size, and the number of measurements were substantially increased, then the distribution would come closer to forming a smooth continuous curve (a frequency curve), perhaps similar to that shown in Figure 3-14.

The frequency curve in Figure 3-15 depicts the distribution of a theoretically infinite set of data, with a theoretically infinitesimal class interval. The frequency distribution that takes the shape similar to that shown in Figure 3-15 is called the normal distribution. Many distributions of measurements of natural objects, biological phenomena, etc. approximate closely the normal distribution. The word "normal" is used to identify rather than to describe the distribution (or curve), and the term "normal distribution" (or "normal curve") does not mean that other distributions (or curves) are abnormal.

Since the normal distribution curve represents the relative frequency, therefore the total area under the curve, being the total of relative frequencies, is equal to 100 percent. Because in a frequency diagram, the frequency is proportional to the area, one can calculate the area within one, two, or three standard deviations and corresponding to these areas frequencies. The area between -1σ and $+1\sigma$ is 68 percent of the total area; this means that in a normal distribution 68 percent of the observations lie within a distance equal to the standard deviation on each side of the mean. Similarly, the distance from -2σ to $+2\sigma$ includes 99 percent of the observations, and the distance from -3σ to $+3\sigma$ includes 99.7 percent of the observations (Fig. 3-16). If one knows the mean and the standard deviation for a particular item, then he can find the area in which a given measurement falls as well as the relative frequency (or probability) of its occurrence. For example, if the mean value and the standard deviation of the QRS duration is 70 and 10 respectively, then the QRS duration of 75 msec. falls inside the interval extending from the mean to the mean + the standard deviation (Fig. 3-17). In terms of relative frequency we may say that such a measurement occurs in 34 percent of all the observations of a normal distribution. The general method of calculating areas (i.e., relative frequencies) is discussed on page 152.

The normal distribution curve is symmetric, with respect to the line drawn perpendicular to the horizontal axis at the mean, which is in the exact center of the curve. If a distribution has a more pronounced "tail" on one side, such as the distribution of Figure 3-18, we say that the distribution is skewed. Thus if a "tail' is on the right, the distribution has positive skewness or it is skewed to the right. Correspondingly, if a distribution has a pronounced "tail" on the left, the distribution has negative skewness or it is skewed to the left.

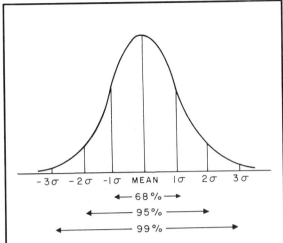

Fig. 3-16. Percentage values of areas (probabilities) under the normal distribution curve.

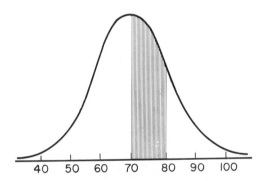

Fig. 3-17. Diagram illustrating the probability of encountering the QRS duration between 70 and 80 msec.

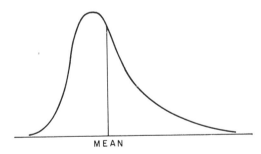

Fig. 3-18. A skewed (to the right) distribution.

NORMAL VECTORCARDIOGRAPHIC VALUES

Physiological Variability

Since no two individuals are precisely alike, the measurement of any vectorcardiographic item yields a collection of different values. The most important factors responsible for the fact that each vectorcardiographic item in normal subjects is spread over considerable range of values, are the following:

1. Constitutional variables such as age, sex, race, weight, chest configuration;
2. Environmental factors such as occupation, physical activity, habitation (including altitude and climate);
3. Condition of patient before taking VCG (exercise, food intake, intake of medications, smoking) and during recording VCG (body position, respiratory position).

A convenient visual presentation of the spread of normal VCG values is obtained by constructing a frequency polygon or histogram. Figure 3-19 shows the observed distribution of the point J amplitude in lead X for 580 normal male subjects, exhibited in the form of a histogram. When the histogram is smoothed, the normal frequency distribution curve can be obtained (Fig. 3-20). For details see page 144.

Normal values of vectorcardiographic items are obtained by a statistical analysis of large samples of normal subjects. Those who are regarded as normal subjects are free from overt cardiovascular disease past or present as well as from diseases such as diabetes mellitus, hypertension, anemia and pulmonary, renal, and peripheral vascular diseases which frequently predispose to cardiovascular disease. However, complete exclusion of cardiovascular pathology in some "normal" cases is impossible and therefore normal values cannot be regarded as absolutely precise.

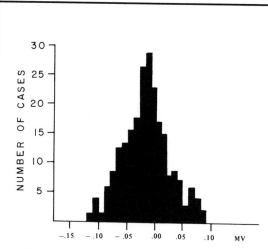

Fig. 3-19. Histogram of the J point amplitude in lead X in 580 normal subjects. Ordinate shows relative frequency.

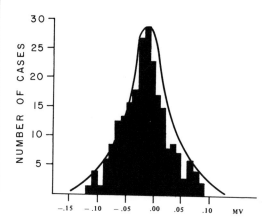

Fig. 3-20. The smoothed curve, showing approximately normal distribution as obtained mathematically from the empirical data represented by the histogram from Figure 3-19.

Normal Limits

Normal limits are arbitrarily defined as the points which enclose 95 percent or 96 percent of the values obtained by measuring a given vectorcardiographic item in normal subjects.

As the lower limit of normal value is taken the mean value minus twice the standard deviation (SD); and as the upper limit of normal value is taken the mean value plus twice the standard deviation. The mean ±2 SD includes about 95 percent of the normal population (Fig. 3-21). These limits can be used only in the case of symmetrical distribution. The distribution of some VCG items, is, however, asymmetrical (i.e., skewed to the right), and in such cases the limits derived from the standard deviations are too narrow at the long end of the distribution and too wide at the short end of the distribution curve.

In the case of asymmetrical distribution, the limits are determined from the 96 percentile ranges. The lower limit is established after eliminating 2 percent of the cases at the "minimal" end of the distribution and the upper limit is established after eliminating 2 percent of the cases at the "maximal" end of the distribution (Fig. 3-22). In the case of symmetrical distribution, the values determined from the SD and the 96 percentile ranges are almost identical.

Because of the great physiological variability of all vectorcardiographic items it is desirable to establish normal limits separately for each sex and for different age groups. The narrower these limits, the greater the chance of accurate differential diagnosis.

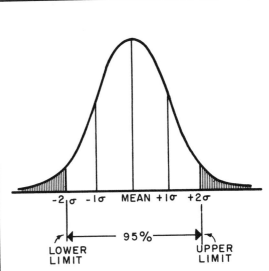

Fig. 3-21. Limits of normal values in the case of normal distribution of a VCG item.

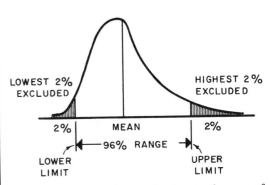

Fig. 3-22. Limits of normal values in the case of assymetrical distribution of a VCG item.

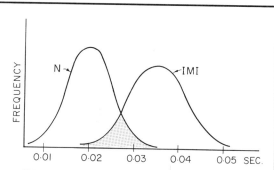

Fig. 3-23. Frequency distribution curve of the Q duration in lead Y in normal population (N) and in patients with inferior myocardial infarction (IMI). Ordinate shows relative frequency within each population.

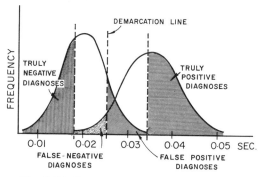

Fig. 3-24. Two overlapping distribution curves when separated by the demarcation (criterion) line yield 4 different regions.

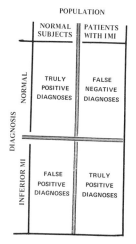

Fig. 3-25. Matrix to illustrate 4 possible regions of classification.

DECISION PROBLEM IN EVALUATING VECTORCARDIOGRAMS

Statistical Technique of Classification

It was mentioned previously that the efficiency of a diagnostic evaluation of VCGs may be improved by analyzing statistical features of VCG items rather than by making decisions on an all-or-none (i.e., yes-or-no), basis. This is illustrated in the following example.

Suppose that the physician finds the Q wave duration in lead Y to be 0.04 sec. He wants to make a hypothesis about the Q being normal or indicating inferior infarction. In order to do this he must know the frequency distribution of the Q wave duration measurements in the normal population and in the population with a well-defined inferior infarction. Those two frequency distributions may be plotted on one scale as shown in Figure 3-23. These frequency distribution curves were plotted on the basis of means and standard deviations (normal p.:M = 0.020, SD = 0.005; infarct p.:M = 0.035, SD = 0.005) assuming a normal distribution. The shaded area in Figure 3-23 represents the overlapping portion of these two distribution curves. This area represents neither exclusively normal population nor exclusively inferior infarction population.

If the physician must decide whether to accept or reject the hypothesis (diagnosis) of the Q wave duration $\geqq$ 0.04 sec. as being evidence of inferior myocardial infarction, he must first decide where to set the demarcation line between the normal population and the population consisting of patients with inferior myocardial infarction. Suppose that this demarcation line has been set at 0.025 sec. (Fig. 3-24). Then the area under the two overlapping curves can be divided into four different regions:

1. Region of truly-positive diagnoses;
2. Region of truly-negative diagnoses;
3. Region of false-positive diagnoses;
4. Region of false-negative diagnoses.

These four possible regions of classification also can be presented in the form of a table (matrix) as shown in Figure 3-25.

A discrimination scale, as shown in Figure 3-24, can be used to determine whether the Q wave duration = 0.04 sec. in lead Y is normal or whether it reflects inferior myocardial infarction. As seen in this figure, the Q wave duration = 0.04 sec. falls in the region of truly-positive diagnoses, so that it should be classified as an infarction Q wave. It is obvious that the correctness of such classification depends to a large extent on a selection of the demarcation line, and this should be decided in such a way as to minimize the total number of misclassifications.

Diagnostic Errors

In most heart diseases, vectorcardiographic items exceed physiological variability (i.e., their frequency distribution differs from that in normal subjects). When the physician is evaluating any VCG item, he must consider the probability of its being a variant of the normal or an evidence of abnormality. It is clear that the probability of being normal is greatest at the median or peak of the distribution curve for a normal population, and decreases from there toward both ends of the distribution curve. Conversely, the probability of being abnormal is greatest at the median or peak of the distribution curve for a given abnormality, and decreases from there toward both ends of this distribution curve. Usually, the distribution of the measurements of a given VCG item in the two populations, normal and diseased, overlaps to some extent, and values are found that can belong to either population (Fig. 3-26). This overlapping leads to the possibility of diagnostic errors.

One type of diagnostic error, as concluding the patient has a disease, when, in fact, he does not, is called a false-positive error (Fig. 3-27). A second type of error is to conclude that the patient does not have the disease, when, in fact, he does. This is a false-negative error (Fig. 3-28). The relative numbers of each type of error depend upon where one sets the normal limits of the population. If the upper limit of normality is set too low, many false-positives are obtained. On the other hand, if the upper limit of normality is set too high, many false-negatives result.

As Figure 3-26 shows, no diagnostic criterion can be entirely satisfactory. However, in some circumstances one may prefer to avoid one type of error at the expense of the other. This preference is usually dictated by considering the relative harm that might result from each type of error, measured in terms of overall well-being of the patient. For example, the harm of calling a patient with angina pectoris normal would be quite great, in view of the serious consequences of failing to treat this disease properly. Consequently, the diagnostic criterion should be set to avoid many false-negative errors. But in this case, many normal persons will be also classified as having angina pectoris (false-positives). However, most physicians feel that it is far more culpable to dismiss a sick patient than to retain a well one. This rule is grounded both on legal proceedings and also on popular sentiment. Although, in the case where the physician suspects that a particular patient has hypochondriacal trends he rather goes to great lengths to avoid a false-positive diagnosis.

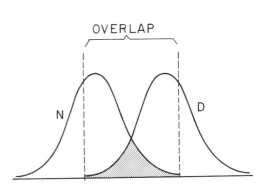

Fig. 3-26. Hypothetical distribution of a VCG item in 2 populations (normal and diseased) showing overlapping.

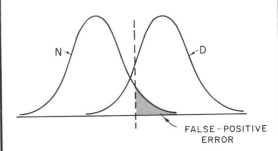

Fig. 3-27. Diagrammatic representation of a false-positive diagnosis (or type I error).

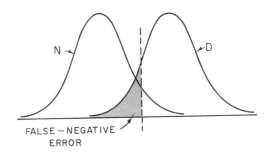

Fig. 3-28. Diagrammatic representation of a false-negative diagnosis (or type II error).

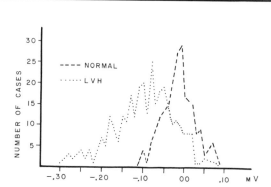

Fig. 3-29. Frequency distribution of the J point amplitude in lead X in normal subjects and in patients with LVH.

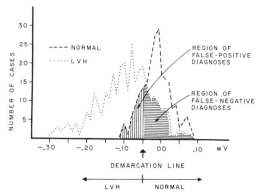

Fig. 3-30. Frequency distribution of the J point amplitude in lead X in normal subjects and in patients with LVH with the demarcation line between them set at −0.05 mv.

Selection of Diagnostic Criteria

The essence of making a diagnostic decision on statistical grounds may be thought of as the selection of diagnostic criterion which minimizes false-negative and false-positive errors, or, in other words, makes a compromise between sensitivity and specificity of the criterion.

To illustrate this point, let us examine Figure 3-29. It shows the distribution of point J amplitude in lead X for normal population and for patients with left ventricular hypertrophy (LVH). It is evident that the upper limit of normal values cannot be chosen as the diagnostic criterion, because it would result in a very high number of false-negative diagnoses. On the other hand, one cannot set the diagnostic criterion close to the mean normal value because it would result in a very high number of false-positive diagnoses. Naturally, one does not want to make either kind of error. Unfortunately, the possibility of doing so cannot often be avoided. Ideally, it is desirable to establish a diagnostic criterion that minimizes missed diagnoses of LVH (false-negative diagnoses) as well as false diagnoses of LVH in normal individuals (false-positive diagnoses). This requirement is approximately met by setting the demarcation line between normal subjects and patients with LVH at −0.05 mv. In such a case only about 20 percent of normal subjects might be diagnosed as having LVH, and at the same time about 30 percent of patients with LVH might be diagnosed as normals (Fig. 3-30).

Although overlapping between normal and diseased populations dictates a compromise in selecting the critical value (diagnostic criterion), there are at least 2 ways to reduce the overlap and decrease the incidence of false diagnoses:

1. The distribution of normal values may be determined separately for different sub-groups of the population which have smaller dispersion than the group as a whole. Comparison of an individual with others of his same age group and body size is an application of this principle.

2. Increasing the sample size is an effective device for reducing diagnostic errors. This is in accord with one's intuition since it is reasonable to conclude that better decisions can be made if more information is available.

Reliability of Diagnostic Criteria

The reliability of a diagnostic criterion in distinguishing normal persons from diseased ones is often defined in terms of sensitivity and specificity. Sensitivity describes the ability of a diagnostic criterion to give a positive diagnosis when the subject examined is truly diseased (i.e., belongs to the diseased population under study). One thus may write

$$\text{Sensitivity (\%)} = \frac{\text{truly-positive diagnoses}}{\text{all members of the diseased population}} \times 100.$$

Specificity describes the ability of a diagnostic criterion to give a negative diagnosis when the subject examined is normal (i.e., belongs to the normal population under study). One may write

$$\text{Specificity (\%)} = \frac{\text{truly-negative diagnoses}}{\text{all members of the normal population}} \times 100.$$

These two terms can be easily appreciated with the help of Figures 3-31 and 3-32. Figure 3-31 shows a hypothetical distribution of the Q duration in two populations, one of normal subjects and one of patients with myocardial infarction. The upper limit of normal has been set at 0.02 sec. (i.e., very low). Thus, this limit (diagnostic criterion), becomes a highly sensitive test for myocardial infarction because all myocardial infarcts are diagnosed. However, this is done at the expense of erroneously suggesting that many normal subjects may have myocardial infarction. If the diagnostic criterion is set at 0.025 sec. this results in lower sensitivity, since not all patients with myocardial infarction are diagnosed correctly. However, in this case, the number of false-positive diagnoses are cut down substantially (Fig. 3-31).

The meaning of specificity is illustrated in Figure 3-32. Here the upper limit of normal Q wave has been set at 0.035 sec. (i.e., very high). Thus, this limit (diagnostic criterion), becomes a highly specific test for myocardial infarction, since no normal cases are diagnosed as infarction. However, this is done at the expense of erroneously suggesting that many patients with myocardial infarction are normal. If the diagnostic criterion is set at 0.03 sec., this results in lower specificity, but at the same time a number of false-negative diagnoses are cut down substantially (Fig. 3-32).

From the above discussion it follows that the gain in sensitivity of a diagnostic criterion is always negated by a loss in specificity, and vice versa. Therefore, the ultimate goal should be the selection of a criterion which minimizes the total number of diagnostic errors (Fig. 3-33).

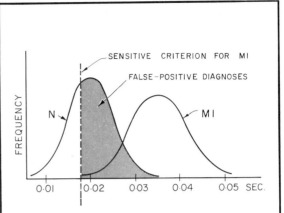

Fig. 3-31. Hypothetical distribution of the Q duration in 2 populations (normal and diseased) showing overlapping. When the upper limit of normal is set low it becomes a highly sensitive test for myocardial infarction.

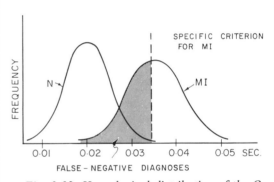

Fig. 3-32. Hypothetical distribution of the Q duration in 2 populations (normal and diseased) showing overlapping. When the upper limit of normal is set high it becomes a highly specific test for myocardial infarction.

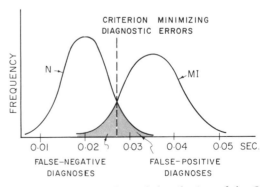

Fig. 3-33. Hypothetical distribution of the Q duration in 2 populations (normal and diseased) showing overlapping. When the upper limit of normal is set intermediate it minimizes both false-positive and false-negative errors.

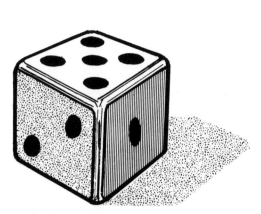

Fig. 3-34. Probability of getting 5 dots in the dice game is about 1/6 or 16 percent.

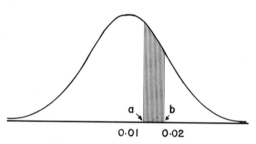

Fig. 3-35. Probability of obtaining an item X being between 0.01 and 0.02 is represented by the shadowed area.

Probability Calculation

More advanced classification procedures, than those outlined above, are based on probability theory. According to this theory, a 1 is assigned to the certain event, a 0 is assigned to the impossible event and any fraction between 0 and 1 is used to measure the uncertainty that a given event will take place. By multiplying such a fraction by 100, one can express the probability of a given event in percentage. For example, if 5 dots appeared 160 times in 1000 tosses, one can assume that the probability of the appearance of 5 dots in the dice game is $\frac{160}{1000}$ or about $\frac{1}{6}$ or 16 percent (Fig. 3-34).

In a case where the frequency distribution of a given VCG item is assumed to be normal, the total area under the curve is by definition equal to 1. Because of this fact, any partial area under the curve can be interpreted as a probability. In order to clarify this statement, let us refer to Figure 3-35, where the probability of obtaining a value between 0.01 and 0.02 is given by the shadowed area. To calculate such a probability, one may use the following formula:

$$P(a < x < b) = \frac{1}{\sqrt{2\pi}} \int_a^b e^{-\frac{1}{2}\left(\frac{x-\mu}{\sigma}\right)} dx$$

where π is the familiar constant whose approximate value is 3.14, e stands for another important constant, the base of the natural system of logarithms whose approximate value is 2.71. In addition to these constants there are two parameters, μ and σ, which stand for the mean value and standard deviation respectively.

In practice, one can obtain such areas (probabilities) under the graph of a normal distribution by means of special tables. These are prepared for the so-called standard normal distribution (i.e., the normal distribution whose mean value equals 0 and whose standard deviation equals 1, Fig. 3-36). In order to use these tables one must convert the units of measurement into standard units by means of the formula

$$z = \frac{x - \mu}{\sigma}.$$

This approach allows one to calculate the probability that a given VCG item comes from the normal population and the probability that it comes from a diseased population. The greater probability points toward the diagnosis. As an example, suppose that Figure 3-37 represents a hypothetical frequency distribution of the R wave amplitude in lead X in the normal population (N) and in the population consisting of patients with well-defined left ventricular hypertrophy (LVH). Now suppose that the R amplitude in lead X obtained from the patient's tracing is 1.5 mv. Then one can calculate the following probabilities:

Probability that R = 1.5 mv belongs to N　　= 10%;
Probability that R = 1.5 mv belongs to LVH = 30%.

Since the sum of these two probabilities must be equal to 1 or 100 percent, (i.e., the event that R = 1.5 mv is either from the normal population or diseased population is certain) then one can write

Probability that R = 1.5 mv belongs to N = 10%
　　　　= 10 ÷ 10 + 30 = 25%;
Probability that R = 1.5 mv belongs to LVH = 30%
　　　　= 30 ÷ 10 + 30 = 75%.

So far, the probability calculation based on one VCG item has been discussed. Of course there is no methodological restriction to calculating the joint probability when many VCG items are under study. Arriving at these calculations is, however, time-consuming and impractical unless it is performed by a computer.

The main difficulty in using mathematical methods to full advantage is the lack of reliable statistics of VCG items in normal and diseased populations. It is hoped that magnetic tape recordings of vectorcardiograms and the use of a computer for their processing may be of great help in solving this problem.

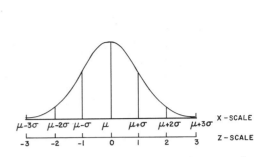

Fig. 3-36. Change of scale in the case of standard normal distribution.

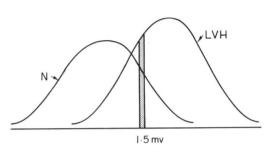

Fig. 3-37. Diagram to illustrate the relative frequency (probability) of obtaining the R peak amplitude in lead X in the neighborhood of 1.5 mv in normal subjects and in patients with LVH.

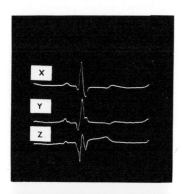

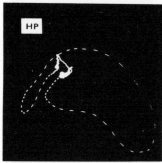

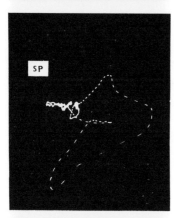

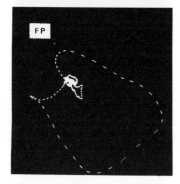

Fig. 3-38. *The VCG record whose report appears on the next page. Recording X, Y, Z: sensitivity 1.0 mV./cm; sweep speed 100 mm./ sec. Recording loops: sensitivity 0.5 mV./cm; dash time 2.5 msec.*

Interpretation of the Vectorcardiogram

VECTORCARDIOGRAM REPORTING SERVICE

Form of the VCG Report

Interpretation of the vectorcardiogram should include the following points:

1. A list of the most important VCG measurements;
2. A brief account of deviations from normal;
3. A statement of the degree of probability that these deviations are produced by pathological factors;
4. A suggestion of clinical diagnosis if this is required by the physician who is in charge of the patient.

The list of VCG measurements may be more or less complete depending mostly on the case being investigated and on local standards. An account of deviations from normal is usually given in terms such as normal VCG, no definitely abnormal findings, suspected abnormal VCG, abnormal VCG.

The information concerning the pathophysiological cause of a deviation is often vague but should be formulated so as not to be misleading to the physician. The fact is that many pathological conditions produce vectorcardiographic patterns that are recognizably abnormal but are not specific for a single disease entity. In such cases it is advisable not to use any definite assessment but simply to state the possible significance of the abnormal findings. Only the physician who is in charge of the patient and knows results of all other examinations can relate VCG changes to underlying disease.

Even though the VCG interpretation is intended merely to provide a suggestion as to the clinical diagnosis, this often requires certain particulars concerning the patient such as age, blood pressure, digitalis medication, chest configuration, weight and eventually others (e.g., sex, pregnancy, chest surgery, clinical problem).

An example of the VCG report form is shown on page 155. Figures in parentheses indicate the lower and upper limits of normal values based on the 96 percent range. The VCG data listed in this report was extracted from the record shown in Figure 3-38.

VECTORCARDIOGRAM
REPORT

Queen's University Teaching Hospital

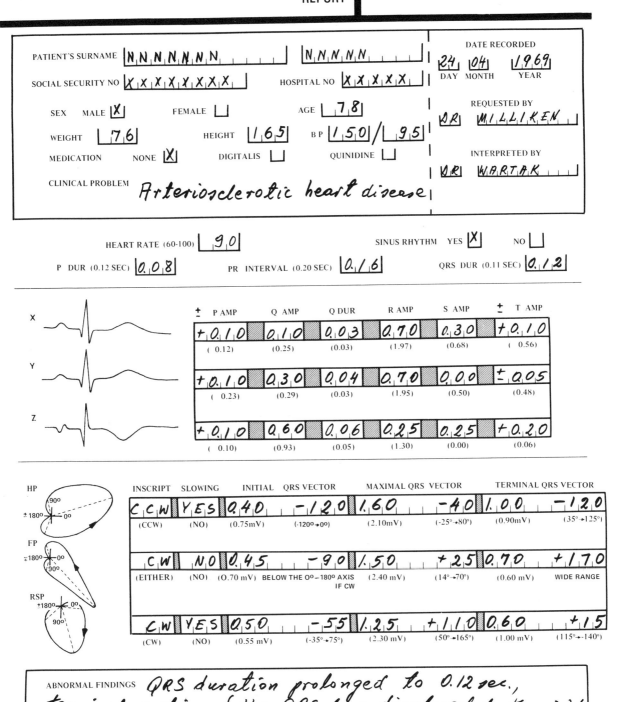

PATIENT'S SURNAME	N N N N N N N	N N N N N		DATE RECORDED

SOCIAL SECURITY NO X X X X X X X X   HOSPITAL NO X X X X X

DATE RECORDED: 24 DAY 04 MONTH 1969 YEAR

SEX MALE X   FEMALE ☐   AGE 7 8

WEIGHT 7 6   HEIGHT 1 6 5   B P 1 5 0 / 9 5

MEDICATION NONE X   DIGITALIS ☐   QUINIDINE ☐

REQUESTED BY DR MILLIKEN

INTERPRETED BY DR WARTAK

CLINICAL PROBLEM Arteriosclerotic heart disease

HEART RATE (60-100) 9 0   SINUS RHYTHM YES X   NO ☐

P DUR (0.12 SEC) 0.0 8   PR INTERVAL (0.20 SEC) 0.1 6   QRS DUR (0.11 SEC) 0.1 2

	± P AMP	Q AMP	Q DUR	R AMP	S AMP	± T AMP
X	+0.10	0.10	0.03	0.70	0.30	+0.10
	(0.12)	(0.25)	(0.03)	(1.97)	(0.68)	(0.56)
Y	+0.10	0.30	0.04	0.70	0.00	±0.05
	(0.23)	(0.29)	(0.03)	(1.95)	(0.50)	(0.48)
Z	+0.10	0.60	0.06	0.25	0.25	+0.20
	(0.10)	(0.93)	(0.05)	(1.30)	(0.00)	(0.06)

	INSCRIPT	SLOWING	INITIAL QRS VECTOR		MAXIMAL QRS VECTOR		TERMINAL QRS VECTOR	
HP	CCW	YES	0.40	-120	1.60	-40	1.00	-120
	(CCW)	(NO)	(0.75mV)	(-120°→0°)	(2.10mV)	(-25°→80°)	(0.90mV)	(35°→125°)
FP	CW	NO	0.45	-90	1.50	+25	0.70	+170
	(EITHER)	(NO)	(0.70 mV) BELOW THE 0°–180° AXIS IF CW		(2.40 mV)	(14°→70°)	(0.60 mV)	WIDE RANGE
RSP	CW	YES	0.50	-55	1.25	+110	0.60	+15
	(CW)	(NO)	(0.55 mV)	(-35°→75°)	(2.30 mV)	(50°→165°)	(1.00 mV)	(115°→-140°)

ABNORMAL FINDINGS QRS duration prolonged to 0.12 sec.,
terminal portion of the QRS loop displaced to the right
and slowly inscribed, initial QRS vectors oriented
COMMENTS superiorly beyond the normal limit

Complete RBBB, probable IMI of uncertain duration

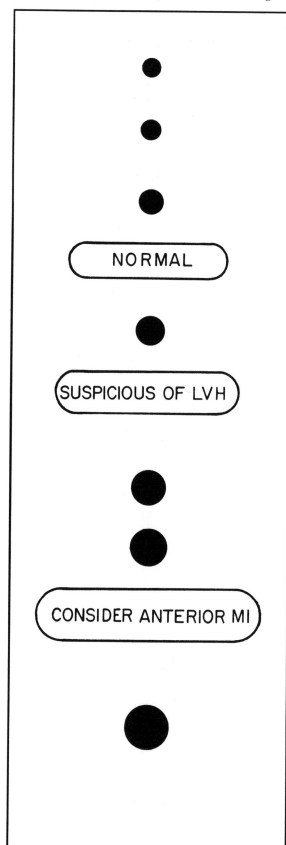

Terminology of the VCG Report

Most vectorcardiographic criteria and diagnostic statements have been standardized. Below are listed terms most frequently used in VCG reports.

X, Y, and Z tracing descriptions

1) amplitude measurements—normal, abnormal, abnormally tall (for a positive deflection), abnormally deep (for a negative deflection), inverted wave, biphasic wave, flat wave (only for the T wave);
2) time measurements—normal, prolonged, shortened, less than . . . , more than . . . ;
3) axis—normal, abnormal, marked LAD, marked RAD, slight LAD, slight RAD, axis of . . . .

Vectorcardiogram loop descriptions

1) loop contour—normal, abnormal, narrow, wide, distorted, showing bite(s), irregular;
2) loop orientation—normal, abnormal, loop pulled (anteriorly, posteriorly, superiorly, inferiorly, leftward, rightward, forward and inferiorly, backward and to the right, leftward and posteriorly), long axis normal, long axis abnormal (see above);
3) loop rotation—clockwise (CW), counterclockwise (CCW), figure-of-eight with initial CW rotation, figure-of-eight with initial CCW rotation, figure-of-eight;
4) loop velocity—normal, initial slowing, mid-portion slowing, terminal slowing, entirely slowing;
5) vector magnitude—normal, increased, decreased, initial (or maximal or terminal) QRS vector magnitude = . . . ;
6) vector orientation—normal, abnormal, anteriorly, posteriorly, superiorly, inferiorly, leftward, rightward, at angle of . . . .

Concluding statements

1) normality—within normal limits, probably normal;
2) questionable normality—borderline, suspicious of . . . ;
3) abnormality—probably abnormal, very probably abnormal, probably . . . , very probably . . . , suggestive of . . . , consider . . . , abnormal VCG consistent with . . . ;
4) indications—suggested 12 lead electrocardiogram, suggested serial vectorcardiogram, suggested post-exercise vectorcardiogram.

CLINICAL VALUE OF VECTORCARDIOGRAM

Limitations of Vectorcardiography

Vectorcardiography must be applied with a full understanding of its limitations. As a rule, a single VCG record is not a sufficient basis for establishing a clinical diagnosis. It can contribute only in a larger or smaller extent to establishing or to confirming a clinical diagnosis. This stems from the fact that the VCG merely records electrical events and they may be disturbed in a similar way by different pathophysiological factors. Thus, a structural or functional impairment of the heart muscle is not automatically reflected in the VCG, and identical tracings are obtained in conditions of completely different etiology and pathogenesis.

Another limitation of vectorcardiography is that it is quite possible to record a normal VCG in the presence of confirmed cardiac disease. On the other hand, abnormal VCGs can be recorded even over considerable periods of time in persons with no recognizable heart disease or impairment of cardiac function.

Still another difficulty that has been experienced in relation to vectorcardiography is that the VCG is subject to influences extraneous to the heart. Particularly sensitive is ST vector and T vector which can be influenced by numerous physiological factors and others (see page 130). It also should be kept in mind that associated pulmonary disease (emphysema, pleural effusion) and previous chest surgery may effect the VCG pattern.

In spite of these limitations, the VCG is an indispensable examination in detecting myocardial infarction, atrial and ventricular hypertrophy, and ventricular conduction defects. The vectorcardiogram is also helpful in controlling effects of certain cardiac medications, particularly digitalis and quinidine and in detecting disturbances in electrolyte metabolism, especially potassium abnormalities.

In some cases, the diagnostic value of vectorcardiographic findings can be considerably increased by repeated recordings at appropriate intervals. This repetition is particularly helpful in such cases as myocardial infarction, pulmonary embolism, myocarditis, etc. (when the course of an illness is followed vectorcardiographically) or in doubtful cases (since a constant finding is usually less significant than one showing sudden changes).

Importance of the Heart Dipole Concept

Vectorcardiography is based on the assumption that the potential distribution at the body surface, produced by the excitation of the heart, can be adequately approximated as a distribution, produced by a dipole generator with a fixed position but time varying magnitude and orientation. The information about the magnitude and orientation of this vector at any instant can be obtained by recording its three orthogonal components by means of the so-called corrected

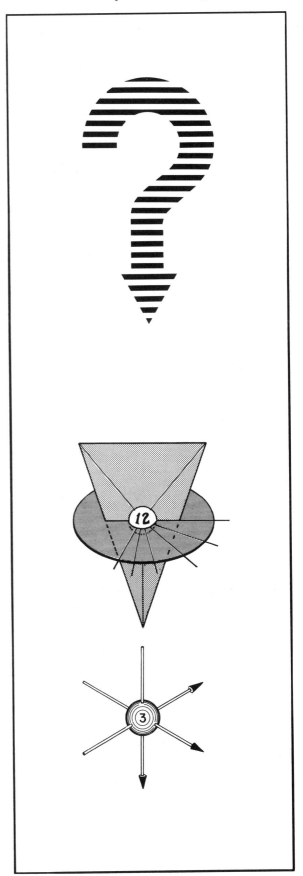

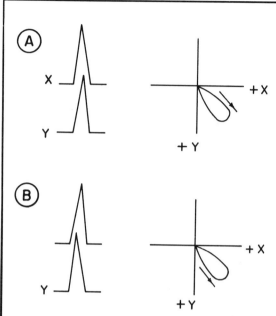

Fig. 3-39. *Diagram illustrating how 2 scalar components of identical configuration but different phase influence the direction of inscription of the vector loop. (A) The peak of R in lead X preceding that in lead Y gives rise to the vector loop inscribed clockwise; (B) The peak of R in lead Y preceding that in lead X gives rise to the vector loop inscribed counterclockwise.*

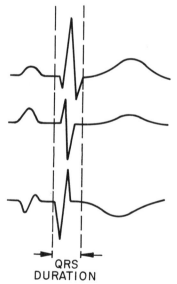

Fig. 3-40. *Diagram to illustrate the principle of measuring of the QRS interval in X, Y, and Z leads.*

orthogonal lead system. The reduction of the number of leads to 3 (as compared to 12 leads in conventional electrocardiography) with probably little, if any, loss of diagnostically important information, simplifies the task of making the analysis because of fewer patterns to be memorized by the physician.

The concept of the heart dipole generator represents a sound biophysical explanation of electrical activity of the heart and makes it possible to use the whole arsenal of mathematical methods for analyzing electrical events of the heart. These methods, especially vector analysis, are extremely useful in understanding most of the electrical phenomena recorded in normal and abnormal hearts.

Another important implication of the heart dipole concept is that, based on it, vectorcardiographic leads provide information that the classical 12 lead system electrocardiograms fail to demonstrate. There are at least two aspects of the cardiac electrical activity that are demonstrated only in the vectorcardiogram. The first involves directional properties of instantaneous heart vectors that can be estimated from the direction of rotation of the vectorcardiographic loop. A difference in the time of onset (phase) of two scalar complexes may produce a totally different direction of the QRS loop and yet not be appreciated on sequentially recorded scalar leads (Fig. 3-39).

The second aspect concerns the accuracy of measuring the ventricular depolarization time. Using the 12 lead system one cannot fully appreciate the exact onset and end of the ventricular depolarization time, since the QRS duration varies from lead to lead depending on the projection of the heart spatial vector on a given lead axis. In vectorcardiography, however, the QRS interval (i.e., the time of the ventricular depolarization) is measured from its earliest commencement in any lead to its latest termination in any lead (Fig. 3-40).

It has been shown that the vectorcardiogram provides valuable diagnostic information in certain conditions in which the 12 lead system electrocardiogram yields only doubtful, if any, information. For example, strictly posterior infarction, very rarely diagnosed in the ECG with any degree of confidence, is a satisfactory vectorcardiographic diagnosis; conduction disturbances are diagnosed more accurately in the VCG; right ventricular hypertrophy is more evident in the VCG; and there are at least four vectorcardiographic patterns underlying that equivocal electrocardiographic finding, rSR' in V_1, each one indicative of a different condition (normal, right ventricular hypertrophy with or without right bundle branch block, and strictly posterior infarction).

It is believed that vectorcardiographic measurements are less influenced by various factors such as location of the heart dipole, the chest configuration, etc. Thus one may expect that discrimination between normals and abnormals is more accurate, since the dispersion of normal values is considerably smaller.

Combined Interpretation of VCG and ECG

The vectorcardiogram and the 12 lead electrocardiogram are different recordings of the same physical phenomenon, namely the electrical activity of the heart. Though much general information about the 12 lead electrocardiogram can be inferred from the vectorcardiogram and vice versa; there are also definite differences between these two methods of recording. Vectorcardiographic leads have been constructed to record three orthogonal components of the heart dipole. However, if one assumes that potential distribution at the body surface cannot be adequately approximated by the heart dipole generator, then the 12 lead system may be superior to the vectorcardiogram in some cases. This is based on the belief that the precordial leads record non-single dipole components, known as a "proximity effect," which are not represented in the orthogonal lead recording.

Another important point is that the 12 lead electrocardiogram has the advantage of providing the precise measurement of time intervals between vectors (P and QRS, P and P, QRS and QRS), a factor which is essential for a proper analysis of cardiac rhythm. When recording vectorcardiograms on the oscilloscope it is usually less convenient to obtain XYZ records including more than a couple of heart cycles.

It is also true that the 12 lead electrocardiogram may be superior to the vectorcardiogram in some cases of combined ventricular hypertrophy. This fact is not surprising, for VCG employs leads that average potential differences picked up from different parts of the body surface, thus equalizing some of the electrical unbalance between the right and left heart.

From the above discussion, it appears that in some cases combined interpretation of the vectorcardiogram and electrocardiogram may increase the diagnostic value of the test.

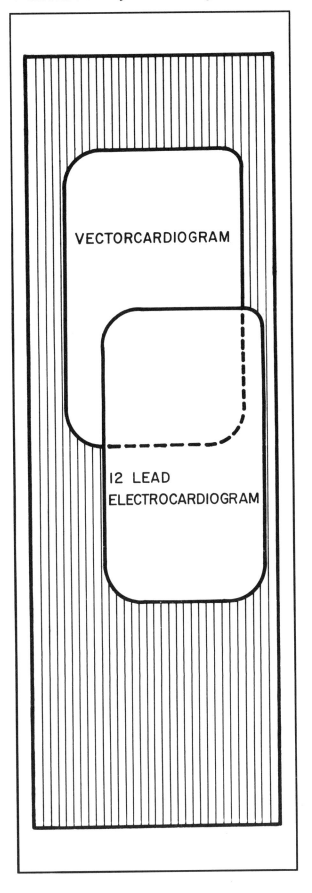

VECTORCARDIOGRAM

12 LEAD ELECTROCARDIOGRAM

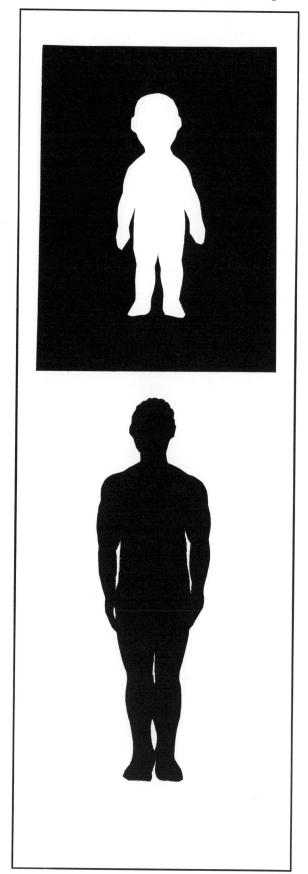

Correlation with Constitutional Variables

Most VCG measurements change with constitutional variables, such as age, race, sex, chest configuration, weight, etc. The understanding of this fact is necessary to appropriately assess the diagnostic significance of a given VCG finding. Below are listed the most important constitutional variables and their effect on VCG items.

Age. Age influences the normal VCG more strongly than any other constitutional variable. The most characteristic change with advancing age is the decrease in magnitude of QRS and ST-T vectors. An average 5 percent decrease in amplitude of QRS vectors, and almost 10 percent decrease in amplitude of ST-T vectors may be allowed for each decade after the age of 30. For example, a value of -0.1 mV for the J point amplitude in lead X is definitely abnormal in subjects below 40, borderline between 40-60, and normal in subjects over 60 years of age. It also should be kept in mind that the vectorcardiogram of normal infants is identical with that of an adult with right ventricular hypertrophy. This "physiologic" right ventricular preponderance (sometimes also called a "juvenile" pattern) may persist up to 10 years of age.

Race. The differences between Negroes and Caucasians include persistence of the "juvenile" pattern in the former, greater prevalence of ST segment elevation with or without tall T wave and higher QRS voltage. Such findings mimic pericarditis, myocardial infarction and acute cor pulmonale. Encountered race differences are attributed to environmental or dietary factors.

Sex. Although there are no obvious differences between the VCGs of males and of females on visual inspection, it has been shown that the magnitudes of the spatial Q, R, and S vectors in males are larger than in females. The most logical explanation for this difference is that females have smaller hearts by weight than males.

Chest configuration. Chest configuration may influence to some extent the VCG. Voltage in lead Z, and in a smaller degree in lead Y, is decreased when the sagittal (anterior-posterior) diameter of the chest is large as compared to the transverse diameter.

Weight. Many of the changes accompanying an increased body weight are similar to those of advancing age (i.e., amplitudes are decreased and the direction of vectors is shifted anteriorly and superiorly).

It is apparent then that the VCG of a given normal individual is influenced by many factors. These factors must be taken into consideration in order to decide how much "variability" or "scatter" may be allowed for normal values of a particular VCG item under given circumstances.

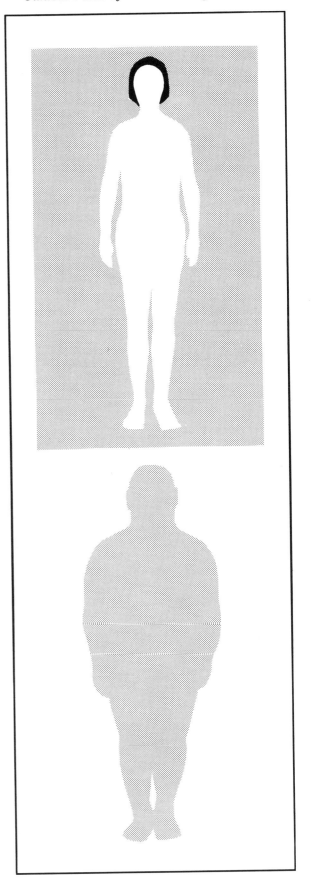

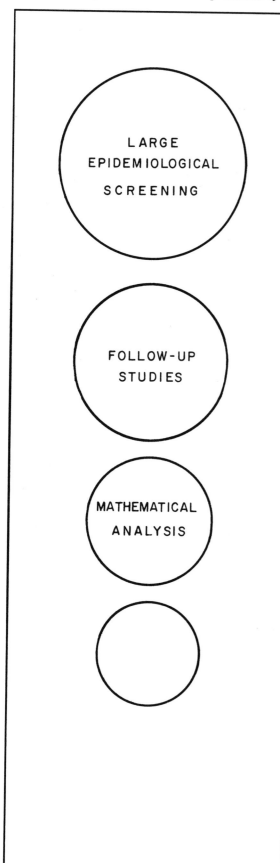

LARGE EPIDEMIOLOGICAL SCREENING

FOLLOW-UP STUDIES

MATHEMATICAL ANALYSIS

Computer Assisted Interpretation of VCGs

AUTOMATED SYSTEM FOR VCG DATA PROCESSING

Objectives of the System

Analysis of the vectorcardiogram performed by the physician is as subjective as any other form of clinical interpretation, and its value depends on his experience, capability of logical reasoning, memory, interest, emotional state, alertness or fatigue, and other factors. Since there are many factors influencing the process of diagnostic evaluation of vectorcardiographic data it is not surprising that there is a considerable variation among cardiologists' interpretations. Careful studies, that have been made to assess the human variability in VCG interpretation, show that cardiologists not only disagree as to whether a given tracing should be labeled as normal or abnormal, but also often fail to agree with their own previous diagnoses on reviewing the records a second time. Hence, some method of eliminating the variations in the VCG interpretation is desirable. The unfailing efficiency and relative objectivity of the computer can be used to accomplish this task.

The reading and interpretation of large numbers of vectorcardiograms can be very tedious, and may lead to boredom and inaccuracy, even among trained cardiologists. By relieving much of this work load, an automated system enables the physician to use his time for the exercise of his highest professional skills.

The opportunity to handle mass data by a computer enables the physician to accomplish large-scale epidemiological screening as well as careful evaluation of serial changes in the electrical activity of the heart. Because of the volume of work involved, serial records are now seldom reviewed.

The unique ability of a computer to perform a large number of numerical computations, in a very short period of time, enables one to apply a variety of mathematical operations for analyzing vectorcardiograms. Some of these mathematical methods are integration, correlation with constitutional variables and discrimination. The integration of the VCG signal aids in the computation of mean vectors, half-area vectors, polar vector, ventricular gradient and others. The correlation between VCG items and constitutional variables enables one to establish more accurate normal values. Mathematical discrimination substantially improves separation between normal and abnormal subjects by performing multivariate analysis, calculating multidimensional probabilities, applying decision rules, etc. If the same set of operations were to be performed by a physician himself it would take several hours or even days for evaluating one vectorcardiogram. A computer does this evaluation within a few seconds.

System Performance

Processing VCG data by a computer involves several operations. First, the VCG data is recorded in a form readable by a computer. This is accomplished by special data acquisition carts which record VCG data on magnetic tape in a frequency modulation (FM) mode (i.e., as an analog signal) or in a digital form. Transmission of the VCG data from the site of recording to the computer center is accomplished by tape playback telephone transmission, or by messenger or by mail delivery of tapes.

Since the analog VCG data is not suitable for handling by most general purpose computers, FM tapes are converted into digital tapes using the so-called analog-to-digital converter. During the conversion, the time continuity of the vectorcardiogram is replaced by a sequence of discrete intervals or samples, which are taken every 2 or 4 milliseconds. The amplitude continuity is removed by assigning to each sample point a numerical value based on its amplitude (Fig. 3-41).

A more advanced system bypasses the need for recording on magnetic tape by providing a direct communication link between the patient and a computer, so that the VCG data is fed directly into the computer's memory. The technician is able to maintain a statement-by-statement conversation with the computer in order to control the flow of data. Using an intricate supervisory program, one also has instant access to the computer and can initiate on-line VCG analysis, regardless what computer program is executing at the time. This system, however, requires very sophisticated interfacing devices and the computer must be equipped with an analog-to-digital converter.

Once the VCG data has been stored in a computer it can be analyzed. This analysis is usually carried out by means of two programs, a pattern recognition program and a diagnosis program. The pattern recognition program identifies the presence of characteristic wave forms in the VCG tracing and measures their amplitude and duration. The diagnostic program classifies the vectorcardiogram as belonging to the normal or abnormal population. The output from the computer is sent to the physician by a messenger, or mail or it is transmitted over a telephone line using TWX telegraphy service. The overall picture of a computer system for processing VCG data is shown in Figure 3-42.

The use of computers in vectorcardiography holds great promise; yet the nature of the computer-oriented contribution must be clearly kept in mind. One must be careful not to have the misapprehension that a computer can do any creative work by itself. All it can do is follow a set of detailed instructions (so-called algorithm) prepared by the physician and/or mathematician and translated into machine readable coding (or program) by the programmer. In general, there is no difficulty in formulating an adequate algorithm for the diagnostic evaluation of vectorcardiograms to be followed by a computer. However, an algorithm for the pattern recognition of vectorcardiograms cannot be adequately formulated at the present time. This failure is due mostly to noise which obscures small waves and smudges the onset and end of most wave form components. The result is an appreciable incidence of errors in recognizing the correct onset and end of the P wave, QRS complex and T wave. Consequently in many cases the value of computer analysis is seriously limited.

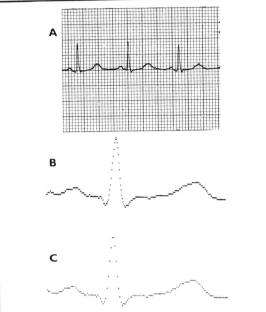

Fig. 3-41. The X lead tracing (A) and its counterpart converted at sampling rate 500 samples per second (B) and 250 samples per second (C). In both cases one millivolt corresponds to 120 conversion units.

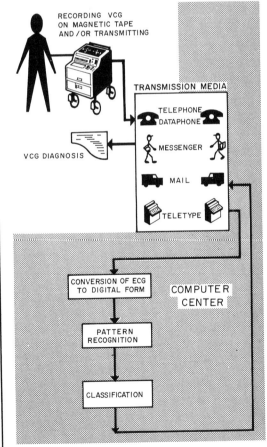

Fig. 3-42. An overall picture of a computer system for processing VCG data.

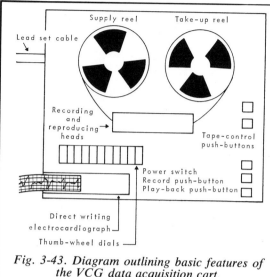

Fig. 3-43. Diagram outlining basic features of the VCG data acquisition cart.

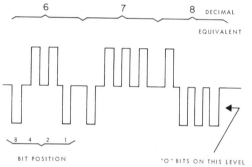

Fig. 3-44. Number 678 as recorded in the binary coded decimal system. Each group of 4 pulses represent a binary code for a decimal digit.

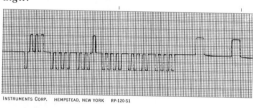

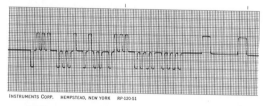

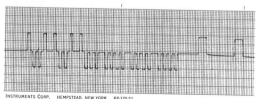

Fig. 3-45. Three channel strip chart showing binary coded data followed by the calibration signal.

VCG DATA ACQUISITION FOR COMPUTER ANALYSIS

Coding the Identification Data

Recording vectorcardiograms for computer analysis is accomplished through special data acquisition "carts". Such devices contain a conventional vectorcardiograph, a patient coding unit and a magnetic tape recorder. The essential features of these instruments are shown in Figure 3-43.

The patient coding unit is used to generate a reliable machine-readable identification of each record. This unit is simply an electromechanical unit employing a number of thumbwheel dials. By rotating each dial, one may pick up any digit from 0 to 9. When the VCG data acquisition console is put in the record mode, the chosen number is then recorded on magnetic tape. The recording is done in a binary coded decimal system (BCD), (i.e., each decimal digit is recorded as a combination of four binary bits). Each bit is defined within its grouping of four binary bits by its position relative to the other three bits and its direction of deflection. The first bit of the grouping of four carries a value of 8, the second a value of 4, the third a value of 2, and the last a value of one. Only upward deflection accepts the value of a bit. Downward deflection converts the value of a particular bit to 0, or in essence rejects it. The summation of all accepted bits in the grouping of four then defines the decimal digit. To simplify reading the code, the time spacing between each digit consisting of four bits is greater than the time between adjacent bits of a digit (Fig. 3-44). For example, a grouping of 4 bits with the first bit deflected down, the second, third and fourth bits deflected up is equivalent to the decimal digit 7. The first bit has a value of 8, but since it is in the downward direction its value is 0. The second bit has a value of 4 in the upward direction and is accepted. The third bit has a value of 2 upward and is accepted. The fourth bit has a value of 1 upward and is accepted. Hence, $0 + 4 + 2 + 1 = 7$.

Binary coded decimal digits as described above are used for recording such data as the patient number, age, weight, and pertinent clinical information. Recording clinical information usually requires the use of a numerical code. For example, sex and race may be coded in the following way: white male—1; white female—2; Negro male—3; Negro female—4; other male—5; other female—6. The identification data and clinical information is shared among the three channels and is recorded, together with the calibration signal. Information that is recorded on magnetic tape also appears on the three-channel strip chart (Fig. 3-45). A chart record may be used for an immediate reading by the physician or for a backup procedure.

Recording VCG Data on Magnetic Tape

Magnetic tape recording is a convenient method for storing the vectorcardiogram in a compact, readily available form for subsequent display or processing by the computer. When the tape recorder is put into playback mode the VCG data is reproduced and may be fed into another piece of equipment (e.g., oscilloscope, analog-to-digital converter, data-phone transmitter). Such a playback can be repeated any number of times without loss of the original information.

Magnetic tape recording of the VCG data can be accomplished either in the analog form or in the digital form. In the former, the VCG data modulates (alters) the frequency of a "carrier oscillator." The frequency of the modulator output is increased proportionately for positive voltage and decreased proportionately for negative voltage. The frequency modulated output is recorded on magnetic tape as a train of magnetic spots which are spaced proportionately to the output signal frequency, or ultimately to the input signal amplitude. This method of recording may be visualized as shown in Figure 3-46. The way the "bit" pulses, the calibration and VCG signals are recorded using FM technique is schematically illustrated in Figure 3-47. During reproduction, the frequency variations in the tape magnetization are detected by the reproducing mechanism and the original signal amplitude is recreated by a demodulator.

Frequency modulation (FM) recording is extremely sensitive to speed variations. Any fluctuation in speed of the tape contributes to the system noise and subsequently to the signal distortion. Also, FM magnetic tapes must be converted into digital form before they can be used as inputs to the computer. These objections may be overcome by the digital technique of recording VCG data. The equipment to accomplish this task has built in an analog-to-digital converter and digital tape recorder in addition to such elements as oscilloscope and/or strip chart recorder and coding unit.

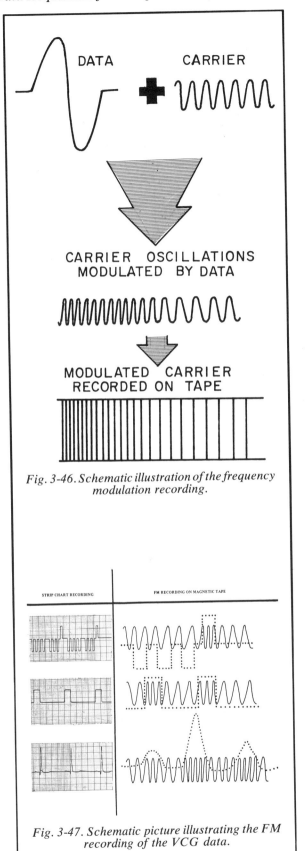

Fig. 3-46. Schematic illustration of the frequency modulation recording.

Fig. 3-47. Schematic picture illustrating the FM recording of the VCG data.

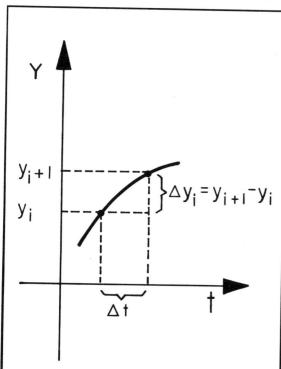

Fig. 3-48. *Geometrical representation of the first difference.*

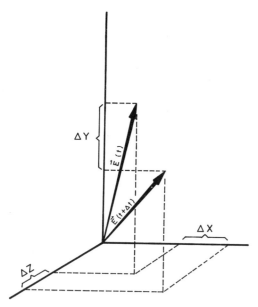

Fig. 3-49. *Diagram to illustrate the concept of the spatial velocity of the heart vector.*

VCG WAVEFORM RECOGNITION BY COMPUTER

Waveform Identification Criteria

One of the major problems of automated analysis of vectorcardiograms is waveform identification. To the human reader the identification of an individual waveform component is based on the wave contour, wave duration and the time of occurrence. In order to have the computer perform VCG pattern recognition, one has to define the contour, onset and end of each wave in mathematical terms (i.e., numerically). This may be accomplished by calculating voltage differences between consecutive data points within a certain interval.

The first difference of voltage between any two consecutive points in the scalar tracing is obtained by subtracting the value of the ith data point from the value of the $(i+1)$th data point (Fig. 3-48). Algebraically this is represented as:

$$\Delta y_i = y_{i+1} - y_i.$$

When the first difference is calculated per unit time Δt, it represents the rate of voltage change (or velocity). Since the three orthogonal leads are considered as scalar components of the heart vector in three-dimensional space, the three voltage changes also can be combined into a vector called spatial velocity (SV) and calculated according to the following formula:

$$SV = \frac{1}{\Delta t} \sqrt{\Delta x_i^2 + \Delta y_i^2 + \Delta z_i^2}$$

where Δx_i, Δy_i, Δz_i are voltage changes in lead X, Y, and Z respectively (Fig. 3-49).

Spatial velocity represents the rate at which the terminus of the heart vector moves in three-dimensional space during the heart cycle. When the magnitude of the spatial velocity vector is plotted against time, one obtains the curve (or function), whose shape is well correlated with the contour of the ECG pattern (Fig. 3-50). A spatial velocity of 7 μ/sec. and greater is usually found only during ventricular depolarization. Spatial velocities below 3 mv/sec. are usually found only during PR and ST segments or TP intervals.

Another criterion which can be used for pattern recognition of the VCG signal is the magnitude of the cardiac spatial vector, which can be calculated from the three orthogonal components X, Y, and Z according to the following formula:

$$M = \sqrt{X^2 + Y^2 + Z^2}$$

where X, Y, and Z represent voltage in lead X, Y, and Z. When the magnitude of the cardiac spatial vector is plotted against time, one obtains the curve or function, so-called spatial magnitude function (SM), whose shape is well correlated with the contour of the ECG pattern (Fig. 3-50). The spatial magnitude function during ventricular depolarization takes on values far above those that occur during the remainder of the heart cycle. Thus the QRS complexes may be recognized when the values of the function rise above an empirically determined threshold and hold that value for longer than 15 msec. In a similar way, the threshold can be set for the P and T waves.

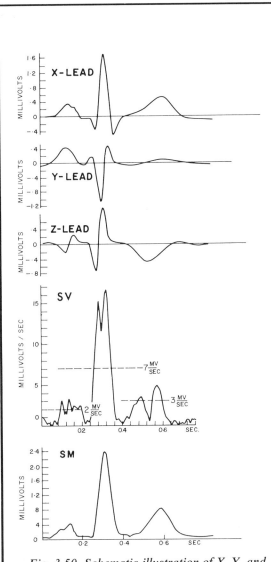

Fig. 3-50. Schematic illustration of X, Y, and Z leads, the spatial velocity (SV) function and the spatial magnitude (SM) function.

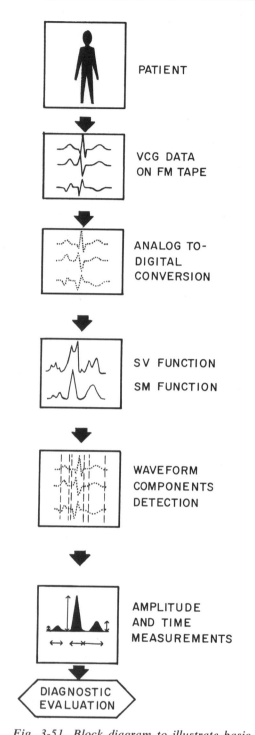

PATIENT

VCG DATA
ON FM TAPE

ANALOG TO-
DIGITAL
CONVERSION

SV FUNCTION

SM FUNCTION

WAVEFORM
COMPONENTS
DETECTION

AMPLITUDE
AND TIME
MEASUREMENTS

DIAGNOSTIC
EVALUATION

Fig. 3-51. Block diagram to illustrate basic procedures involved in the VCG pattern recognition.

Locating Waveform Components

The VCG pattern recognition is schematically depicted in Figure 3-51. At the beginning, the VCG data from the analog tape is converted into numerical form. When this operation is completed the computer calculates two functions, namely spatial velocity and spatial magnitude of the cardiac vector, which then are used for locating QRS complexes, P waves and T waves.

A summary flowchart of the procedure for defining the onset and end of the VCG waveform components is given in Figure 3-52. After having calculated spatial magnitude (SM) and spatial velocity (SV) for all points, the program examines SM values until a point is reached where the value is above the threshold level (L). This point is labeled as i Max and it defines location of the QRS complex. The program then examines SV values for points preceding i Max, and for points following i Max in order to find the points at which the spatial velocity stays below 7 μV/sec. for a period of time (approximately 8 msec.). These points are used to locate the onset and end of the QRS complex. Having established the onset and end of the QRS complex, the program locates the next QRS complex and determines its onset and end. After having examined the whole tracing for the presence of QRS complexes, the program then locates the P wave and T wave between two consecutive QRS complexes.

The P wave is found by searching for a sequence of points where the spatial velocity exceeds 3 μV/sec. This search region extends from the onset of the QRS complex to a point approximately halfway between two adjacent QRS complexes. The T wave is located in the region from the end of the QRS complex to the beginning of the P wave in the next cycle. Determination of the T wave is based on the same criteria as those used for the P wave determination; but the T wave determination goes forward, while in the case of the P wave, it goes backward. Onset of either P wave or T wave in the appropriate interval is determined as the first point on the SV function whose value emerges from the noise level and is followed by points for which the SM function increases with time. The end of either T wave or P wave is determined as the last point on the SV function whose value emerges from the noise level and is preceded by points, for which the SM function decreased with time. The noise level may be determined by averaging values of the SV function over a range of about 20 msec. backward from the beginning of the QRS complex. In most cases the spatial velocity found within the noise level is below 3 mV/sec.

After the time location for the onset and end of each waveform component is ascertained in X, Y, and Z leads, the program calculates the instantaneous vectors in the frontal, horizontal and left sagittal planes. The instantaneous planar vectors are summed over desirable time intervals, and the magnitude and orientation of these mean vectors are used later for diagnostic evaluation. These vectors depicted in Figure 3-53, represent the initial and terminal atrial depolarization, the initial, main, and terminal portions of ventricular depolarization, and three equal portions of ventricular depolarization.

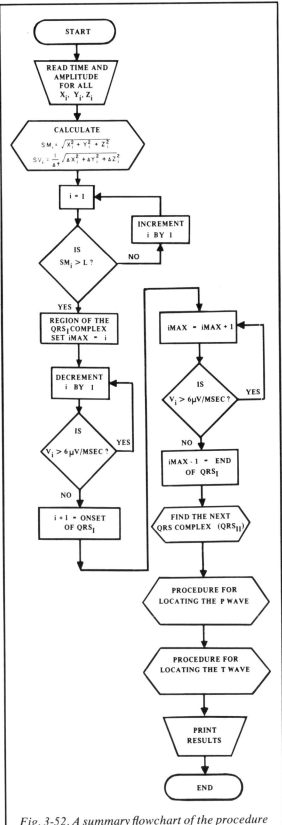

Fig. 3-52. A summary flowchart of the procedure for VCG pattern recognition.

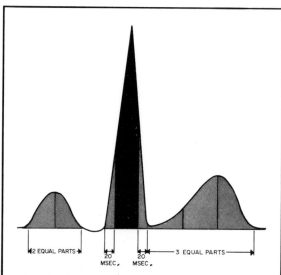

Fig. 3-53. *Diagram depicting mean cardiac vectors that are used for diagnostic evaluation.*

DECISION TABLE FORM		
STUB	ENTRY	
	RULE NUMBER	
	1 2 3 . . . . . . E	

CONDITIONS

EACH ROW CONTAINS A CONDITION TO BE TESTED	EACH COLUMN IS A PARTICULAR COMBINATION OF TESTS TO BE SATISFIED

ACTIONS

EACH ROW LISTS AN ACTION TO BE TAKEN	EACH COLUMN CONTAINS ACTIONS DICTATED BY TEST COMBINATION SATISFIED ABOVE

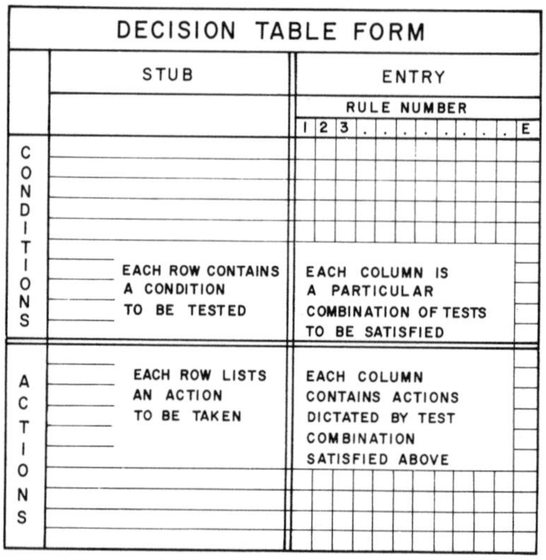

Fig. 3-54. *The skeleton outline of a decision table.*

VCG DIAGNOSIS BY COMPUTER

Decision Tables Technique

The use of a computer for diagnosing vectorcardiograms requires a detailed description of the sequence in which the tracing is to be evaluated. The physician usually does not follow a strictly defined sequence in evaluating vectorcardiograms, because he can analyze many items almost simultaneously, evaluate each item in the light of the overall appearance of the tracing and reevaluate his preliminary assessment. But it is not the case with a computer which operates in a serial mode rather than in a parallel one. Computer needs to be told that item A must be evaluated first and, depending on the result, the next step must be such and such, etc. Thus, it is obvious that in order to use a computer for diagnosing vectorcardiograms one has to provide detailed logic for diagnostic evaluation.

The logic involved in diagnostic evaluation of the VCG data is best expressed in the form of decision trees or decision tables. The decision tree structure and how it can be used for diagnosing VCG data has been described on page 138. While the decision tree depicts the diagnostic process in sequential steps, the decision table depicts it in vertical, parallel columns, so that similarities and differences among various columns can be much better appreciated.

The structure of the decision table is straightforward. Each table is divided into four quadrants by double lines (Fig. 3-54). The vertical double line separates the stub on the left from the entry which appears on the right. The horizontal double line separates conditions from actions. Thus the upper left quadrant contains a series of conditions (questions) which are to be tested while the lower left quadrant describes the actions to be taken depending on the outcome of these tests.

Each column in the entry makes up a decision rule. A decision rule may consist of at least 2 of the 4 entries shown in Figure 3-55. Rules are sequence-numbered for convenience, as shown in Figure 3-54. The set of conditions specified by each rule must be unique so as to avoid ambiguity. Equivalent sets of conditions leading to different actions are erroneous. The converse—different conditions leading to the same action—is permissible and even may be desirable.

Any rules not specified or implied in the table are assumed to be part of the ELSE-RULE. This rule is the column farthest right which contains no entries in the condition part of the table. It specifies the actions to be taken if none of the rules is satisfied.

Mechanics of Using Decision Tables

Decision tables are excellent means of describing the relationship between VCG items and VCG diagnostic categories, which may be thought of as a sequence of statements that fit the pattern:

> If . . . and if . . . and if . . .
> (conditions are true),
> then . . . and . . . and . . .
> (actions are to be taken).

A complete process of diagnosing vectorcardiographic patterns has been depicted in the decision table shown in Figure 3-56. The first condition row in this table checks to see whether the initial QRS vector is oriented anteriorly. The outcome NO (N) of this test appears in rule No. 1. The outcome YES (Y) of the first test appears in all the rest of the rules. In rule No. 3 no entry is made for the fourth, sixth and ninth conditions because they are immaterial for this rule. A YES (Y) entry is made for the first and the third conditions and a NO (N) entry is made for the second, fifth, seventh and eighth conditions. The action specified for rule No. 3 is action Row 3 which says: "Lateral myocardial infarction."

For an illustration of the evaluating procedure, suppose that one enters the VCG diagnosis table with the following items extracted from the patient's record: QRS duration equals 0.10 sec., PR interval equals 0.14 sec., initial (0-30 msec.) QRS vectors oriented anteriorly, inferiorly and rightward, the maximal QRS vector in the horizontal plane measures 1.8 mV, the mean QRS vector in the frontal plane directed at 85°. Because initial QRS vectors are directed anteriorly, the first condition in the first rule is not satisfied and checking is moved to the second rule. In this rule the first condition is satisfied, but the second condition is not, so the checking is moved to the third table. This rule matches for the patient data. The action for the third rule is listed in action Row 3. Having readied the first rule, which matches for the patient data, one may ignore any further columns to the right. If no rule in this table were satisfied, then the ELSE RULE would come into action.

By use of decision tables the physician can synthesize useful algorithm for the VCG data analysis, which subsequently can be translated into machine readable coding and executed by the computer.

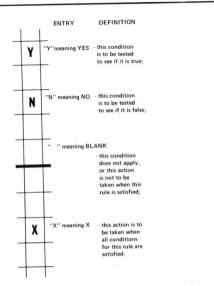

Fig. 3-55. *Four different entries used in decision tables.*

DECISION TABLE	TABLE NAME VCG DIAGNOSIS	RULE NUMBER										
		1	2	3	4	5	6	7	8	9	10	E
INITIAL QRS VECTORS DIRECTED ANTERIORLY		N	Y	Y	Y			Y	Y	Y	Y	
INITIAL QRS VECTORS DIRECTED SUPERIORLY			Y	N	N	N	N	N	N	N	N	
INITIAL QRS VECTORS DIRECTED RIGHTWARD				Y	N						N	
MAX QRS VECTOR IN HP AT -15° OR BELOW					Y							
QRS INTERVAL ≥ 0.12 SEC		N		N	N	Y	Y	N	N		N	
PR INTERVAL > 0.12 SEC						N	Y	Y	Y			
MAX QRS VECTOR IN HP ≥ 2.2 MV				N	N			Y	N	N		
MEAN QRS VECTOR IN FP AT 110° OR MORE				N	N				Y	Y	N	
MAX QRS VECTOR IN HP ≥ 1.5 MV										N	Y	
ANTERIOR MI		x										
INFERIOR MI			x									
LATERAL MI				x								
POSTERIOR MI					x							
WPW SYNDROME						x						
VENTRICULAR CONDUCTION DEFECT							x					
LEFT VENTRICULAR HYPERTROPHY								x				
RIGHT VENTRICULAR HYPERTROPHY									x			
BIVENTRICULAR HYPERTROPHY										x		
WITHIN NORMAL LIMITS											x	
UNDETERMINED PATTERN												x

Fig. 3-56. *Decision table for diagnosing vectorcardiograms.*

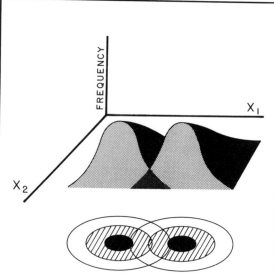

Fig. 3-57. Diagram depicting the joint probability density in 2-dimensional space for 2 hypothetical populations (normal and diseased).

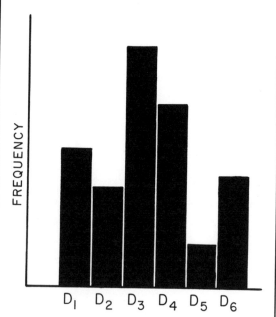

Fig. 3-58. Diagram to illustrate the prevalence of diagnostic categories.

Calculating the Joint Probability

Another approach to computerizing the vectorcardiographic diagnosis is based on probability calculus. An introduction to this subject has been given on page 152.

The joint probability density function of n VCG items can be calculated using the following formula:

$$P(X_1, X_2, \cdots, X_n) = \frac{|A|^{\frac{1}{2}}}{(2\pi)^n} e^{-\frac{1}{2}\sum_{j=1}^{n}\sum_{k=1}^{n} a_{jk}(X_j-\overline{X}_j)(X_k-\overline{X}_k)}$$

where $|A|$ is the determinant of the inverted covariance matrix, a_{jk} is the element of the jth row and the kth column of the inverted covariance matrix, and $\overline{X}$ is the mean of a corresponding VCG item.

The joint probability density of a particular set of n VCG items can be visualized as a point within an ellipsoid of a specified frequency in a hypothetical n-dimensional space. Such a space cannot be visualized, but one can get the idea of this technique from the picture in two-dimensional space (Fig. 3-57).

If, in addition, the prevalence of diagnostic categories (diseases) is known, one may calculate the probability of the incidence of specified diseases given a particular set of VCG items (Fig. 3-58). This can be accomplished according to the Bayes theorem given as

$$P(D_i/S) = C \ P(S/D_i) \ P(D_i)$$

where $P(D_i/S)$ is the probability that the patient has disease D_i when a particular set of vectorcardiographic findings S is observed; $P(S/D_i)$ is the probability of occurrence of a particular set of vectorcardiographic findings (S), given a population with disease D_i; and $P(D_i)$ is the a priori probability of having disease D_i for the population of which the patient is a member. In other words, $P(D_i)$ is a statement of the prevalence of disease D_i expressed as its frequency in the population from which the patient is considered to be a sample, such as a hospital population, or the population at large, or some other population. Symbol C is a normalizing factor such that $\Sigma \ P(D_i/S) = 1$, thus

$$C = 1 \div \sum_{i=1}^{n} P(S/D_i) \ P(D_i)$$

where n is the number of diseases concerned.

Unfortunately, the use of the Bayes theorem is limited by the fact that in present medical situation $P(D_i)$ and $P(S/D_i)$ are not readily available, because of lack of good data.

Part 4
Bibliography

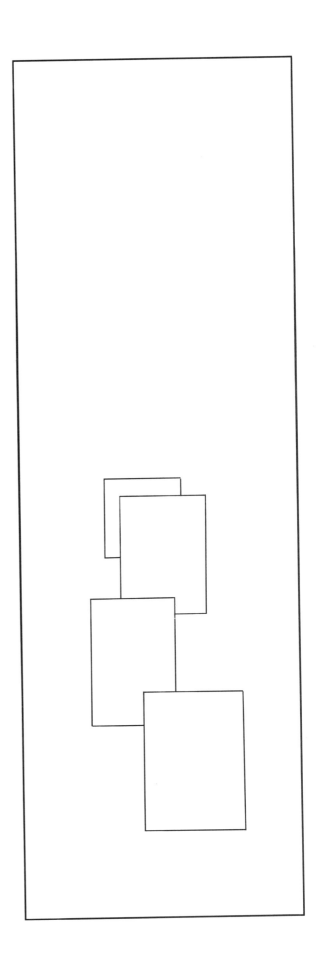

Bibliography

Electrical activity of the heart

Attwood, S. S.: Electric and Magnetic Fields. New York, Dover Publications, 1967.

Bennet, G. A.: Electricity and Modern Physics. London, Edward Arnold & Co., 1968.

Briller, S. A.: Ionic exchanges and cardiac action potential in relation to electrocardiogram. Progr. Cardiovasc. Dis., 2:207, 1960.

Geselowitz, D. B.: Dipole theory in electrocardiography. Am. J. Cardiol., 14:301, 1964.

Geselowitz, D. B.: Multipole representation for an equivalent cardiac generator. Proc. IRE, 48:75, 1960.

Hoffman, B. F., and Cranefield, P. F.: Electro-physiology of the Heart. New York, McGraw-Hill, 1960.

Johnston, F. D.: The spread of currents and distribution of potential in homogeneous volume conductors. Ann. N. Y. Acad. Sci., 65:963, 1957.

Nachmansohn, D.: Generation of bioelectric potentials. Circ. Res., 3:429, 1955.

Page, E.: The electrical potential difference across the cell membrane of heart muscle. Circulation, 26:582, 1962.

Schaffer, A.: The body as a volume conductor. Am. Heart J., 51:588, 1956.

Scher, A. M.: The sequence of ventricular excitation. Am. J. Cardiol., 14:294, 1964.

Taccardi, B.: Distribution of heart potentials on the thoracic surface of normal human subjects. Circulation Res., 12:341, 1963.

Weidmann, S.: Cardiac membrane potentials. J. Physiol., 127:213, 1955.

Yarwood, J., and Close, K. J.: Introductory Electricity and Atomic Physics, London, Longmans, 1965.

Vector representation of the heart electrical forces

Bayley, R. H.: Biophysical Principles of Electrocardiography. New York, Paul B. Hoeber, 1958.

Boutkan, J.: Vectorcardiography. Physical Bases and Clinical Practice. Eindhoven, Centrex Publishing, 1965.

Burger, H. C., and Vaane, J. P.: A criterion characterizing the orientation of a vectorcardiogram in space. Am. Heart J., 56:32, 1958.

Goldberger, E.: How to Interpret Electrocardiograms in Terms of Vectors. Springfield, Ill., Charles C Thomas, 1968.

Grant, R. P.: Clinical Electrocardiography. The Spatial Vector Approach. New York, McGraw-Hill, 1957.

Grishman, A.: Spatial Vectorcardiography. In Luisada, A. A. (ed.): Examination of the Cardiac Patient. New York, McGraw-Hill, 1965.

Miller, K. S.: A Short Course in Vector Analysis. Charles E. Merrill Books, Inc., 1966.

Okomoto, N., and Simonson, E.: Separation of normal and abnormal vectorcardiograms. Am. J. Cardiol., 18:682, 1966.

Penaloza, D., and Tranchesi, J.: The three main vectors of the ventricular activation process in the normal human heart. I. Its significance. Am. Heart J., 49:51, 1955.

Schwartz, M., Green, S., and Rutledge, W. A.: Vector Analysis. New York, Harper & Brothers, 1960.

Lead systems for recording electrical activity of the heart

Burger, H. C., and van Milaan, J. B.: Heart vector and leads. I. Brit. Heart J., 8:157, 1946. II. Ibid., 9:154, 1957. III. Ibid., 10:229, 1948.

Frank, E.: General theory of heart-vector projection. Circ. Res., 2:258, 1954.

Frank, E.: The image surface of a homogeneous torso. Am. Heart J., 47:757, 1955.

Frank, E.: An accurate clinically practical system for spatial vectorcardiography. Circulation, 13:737, 1956.

Goldberger, E.: A simple indifferent electrocardiographic electrode of zero potential and a technique of obtaining augmented, unipolar leads. Am. Heart J., 23:483, 1942.

Goldberger, E.: Unipolar Lead Electrocardiography and Vectorcardiography. Philadelphia, Lea & Febiger, 1953.

Goldberger, E.: Vector leads. Am. J. Cardiol., 6:997, 1960.

Helm, R. A.: Mathematical methods for analyzing leads. Am. Heart J., 57:149, 1959.

Helm, R. A., and Chou, T-C.: Electrocardiographic leads. Am. J. Cardiol., 14:317, 1964.

Langner, P. H., Jr.: An octaxial reference system derived from a nonequilateral triangle for frontal plane vectorcardiography. Am. Heart J., 49:696, 1955.

Langner, P. H., Jr., Okada, R. H., Moore, S. R., and Fies, H. L.: Comparison of four orthogonal systems of vectorcardiography. Circulation, 17:46, 1958.

McFee, R., and Johnston, F. D.: Electrocardiographic leads. I. Introduction. Circulation, 8:554, 1953. II. Analysis. Ibid., 9:255, 1954. III. Synthesis. Ibid., 9:868, 1954.

McFee, R., and Parungao, A.: An orthogonal lead system for clinical electrocardiography. Am. Heart J., 62:93, 1961.

Schmitt, O.: Lead vectors and transfer impedance. Ann. N.Y. Acad. Sci., 65:1092, 1957.

Simonson, E.: Vectorcardiographic leads: historical perspectives. In Proc. Long Island Jewish Hosp. Symposium Vectorcardiography. North-Holland Publishing Company, 1966.

Wilson, F. N., Johnston, F. D., and Kossmann, C. E.: The substitution of a tetrahedron for the Einthoven triangle. Am. Heart J., 33:594, 1947.

Wilson, F. N., Johnston, F. D., MacLeod, A. G., and Barker, P. S.: Electrocardiograms that represent the potential variations of a single electrode. Am. Heart J., 9:447, 1934.

Instruments recording electrical activity of the heart

Brinberg, L.: A three-dimensional display of vectorcardiograms. Cardiov. Res., 3:329, 1969.

Dower, G. E., Horn, H. E., and Ziegler, W. G.: The polarocardiograph. Terminology and normal findings. Am. Heart J., 69:355, 1965.

Lamb, L. E.: Electrocardiography and Vectorcardiography. Philadelphia, W. B. Saunders, 1965.

Laufberger, V.: Spatiocardiography. Textbook and Atlas. Prague, Publishing House of the Czechoslovak Academy of Sciences, 1964.

Massie, E., and Walsh, T. Y.: Clinical Vectorcardiography and Electrocardiography. Chicago, Year Book Publishers, 1960.

Moore, A. D., Harding, P., and Dower, G. E.: The polarcardiograph. An analogue computer that provides spherical polar coordinates of the heart vector. Am. Heart J., *64*:382, 1962.

Schmitt, O. H.: Cathode-ray presentation of three-dimensional data. J. Appl. Physics, *18*:819, 1947.

Methods of analyzing electrical activity of the heart

Abildskov, J. A., Ingerson, W. E., and Hisley, B. L.: A linear time scale for spatial vectorcardiographic data. Circulation, *14*:556, 1956.

Abildskov, J. A., and Wilkinson, R. S., Jr.: The relation of precordial and orthogonal leads. Circulation, *27*:58, 1963.

Brinberg, L.: Quantitative Vector Electrocardiography. Baltimore, Waverly Press, 1960.

Chou, T-C., and Helm, R. A.: Clinical Vectorcardiography. New York, Grune & Stratton, 1967.

Friebrun, J. L., Isaacs, J. H., and Griffith, G. C.: The vectorelectrocardiogram. A simple method of recording and interpreting the spatial electrical field of the heart. Am. J. Cardiol., *5*:390, 1960.

Goldberger, E.: Electrovectorcardiography. A simple method of studying vectorcardiography, using the conventional electrocardiogram. Am. J. Cardiol., *3*:124, 1959.

Howard, F. H.: A method for the construction of the vectorcardiogram from the Einthoven electrocardiogram. Am. Heart J., *31*:191, 1946.

Helm, R. A., and Fowler, N. O., Jr.: A simplified method for determining the angle between two spatial vectors. Am. Heart J., *45*:835, 1953.

Helm, R. A.: Vectorcardiographic notation. Circulation, *13*:581, 1956.

Report of Committee on Electrocardiography, American Heart Association. Recommendation for standardization of leads and specifications for instruments in electrocardiography and vectorcardiography. Circulation, *35*:583, 1967.

Winsor, T., Sibley, A. E., Fisher, E. K., *et al.*: An approach to vectorcardiography. The rectilinear vectorcardiogram. Am. J. Cardiol., *18*:651, 1966.

Witham, A. C.: Quantitation of the vectorcardiogram. Am. Heart J., *72*:284, 1966.

Normal patterns of electrical activity of the heart

Beswick, F. W., *et al.*: Normal spatial orthogonal vectorcardiographic data. Am. J. Cardiol., *16*:321, 1965.

Bristow, J. D.: A study of the normal Frank vectorcardiogram. Am. Heart J., *61*:242, 1961.

Chou, T-C., and Helm, R. A.: Clinical Vectorcardiography. New York, Grune & Stratton, 1967.

Draper, H. W., Peffer, C. J., Stallman, F. W., *et al.*: The corrected orthogonal electrocardiogram and vectorcardiogram in 510 normal men (Frank lead system). Circulation, *30*:853, 1964.

Estes, E. H.: Electrocardiography and vectorcardiography.

In Hurst, J. W., and Logue, R. B. (ed.): The Heart. McGraw-Hill, 1966.

Grant, R. P.: Clinical electrocardiography. The Spatial Vector Approach. New York, McGraw-Hill, 1957.

Gunther, L., and Graf, W. S.: The normal adult spatial vectorcardiogram. Am. J. Cardiol., *15*:656, 1965.

Milnor, W. R.: The normal vectorcardiogram and a system for the classification of vectorcardiographic abnormalities. Circulation, *16*:95, 1957.

McCall, B. W., Wallace, A. G., and Estes, E. H.: Characteristics of the normal vectorcardiogram recorded with the Frank lead system. Am. J. Cardiol., *10*:514, 1962.

Wartak, J.: Electrocardiographic Tables. Montreal, R. E. Squibb Company, 1970.

Abnormal patterns of electrical activity of the heart

Chou, T-C., and Helm, R. A.: Clinical Vectorcardiography. New York, Grune & Stratton, 1967.

Dimond, E. G.: Electrocardiography and Vectorcardiography. Boston, Little, Brown and Company, 1967.

Grant, R. P.: Clinical Electrocardiography. The Spatial Vector Approach. New York, McGraw-Hill, 1957.

Massie, E., and Walsh, T. J.: Clinical Vectorcardiography and Electrocardiography. Chicago, Year Book Publishers, 1960.

Sodi-Pallares, D., and Calder, R. M.: New Bases of Electrocardiography. St. Louis, C. V. Mosby, 1956.

Uhley, H. N.: Vector Electrocardiography. Philadelphia, J. B. Lippincott, 1962.

Hypertrophy of the heart muscle

Bristow, J. D., Porter, G. A., and Griswold, H. E.: Observations with the Frank system of vectorcardiography in left ventricular hypertrophy. Am. Heart J., *62*:621, 1961.

Cabrera, E., and Gaxiola, A.: A critical reevaluation of systolic and diastolic overloading patterns. Prog. Cardiov. Dis., *2*:219, 1959.

Cabrera, E., and Gaxiola, A.: Diagnostic contribution of the vectorcardiogram in hemodynamic overloading of the heart. Am. Heart J., *60*:296, 1960.

Castellanos, A., Hernandez, F. A., Lemberg, L., *et al.*: The vectorcardiographic criteria of hemodynamical overloadings in congenital heart disease. Cardiologia, *44*:392, 1964.

Chou, T-C., and Helm, R. A.: The pseudo P pulmonale. Circulation, *32*:96, 1965.

Chou, T-C., and Helm, R. A.: Clinical Vectorcardiography. New York, Grune & Stratton, 1967.

Cueto, J., Toshima, H., Armijo, G., *et al.*: Vectorcardiographic studies in acquired valvular disease with reference to the diagnosis of right ventricular hypertrophy. Circulation, *33*:588, 1966.

Dack, S.: The electrocardiogram and vectorcardiogram in ventricular septal defect. Am. J. Cardiol., *5*:199, 1960.

Fowler, N. O., and Helm, R. A.: The spatial QRS loop in right ventricular hypertrophy with special reference to the initial component. Circulation, *7*:573, 1953.

Hugenholtz, P. G., and Gamboa, R.: Effect of chronically increased ventricular pressure on electrical forces of the heart. A correlation between hemodynamic and vectorcardiographic data (Frank system) in 90 patients with aortic or pulmonic stenosis. Circulation, *30*:511, 1964.

Hugenholtz, P. G., Ellison, R. C., and Miettinen, O. S.: Spatial voltages in the assessment of left ventricular hypertrophy (Frank system), J. Electrocardiol., *1*:77, 1968.

Khoury, G. H., DuShane, J. W., and Ongley, P. A.: The preoperative and postoperative vectorcardiogram in tetralogy of Fallot. Circulation, *31*:85, 1965.

Lasser, R. P., Borun, E. R., and Grishman, A.: Spatial vectorcardiography: right ventricular hypertrophy as seen in congenital heart disease. VII. Am. Heart J., *42*:370, 1951.

Mazzoleni, A., Wolff, R. and L.: The vectorcardiogram in left ventricular hypertrophy. Am. Heart J., *58*:648, 1959.

McCaughan, D., Koroxenidis, G. T., Hopff, L. G., and Williams, C.: New vectorcardiographic criteria for the diagnosis of acquired right ventricular hypertrophy: Comparison with standard electrocardiographic criteria (P). Circulation, *28*:766, 1963.

Milnor, W. R.: Electrocardiogram and vectorcardiogram in right ventricular hypertrophy and right bundle branch block. Circulation, *16*:348, 1957.

Murata, K., Kurihara, H., Matsushita, S., *et al.*: Significance of T-loop change in vectorcardiographic diagnosis of left ventricular hypertrophy. Am. Heart J., *73*:49, 1967.

Murata, K., Kurihara, H., Hosoda, H., *et al.*: Frank lead vectorcardiogram in left ventricular hypertrophy. Jap. Heart J., *5*:543, 1964.

Richman, J. L., and Wolff, L.: The spatial vectorcardiogram in congenital heart disease and right ventricular hypertrophy. Am. Heart J., *50*:85, 1955.

Romhilt, D. W., Greenfield, J. C., and Estes, E. H.: Vectorcardiographic diagnosis of left ventricular hypertrophy. Circulation, *37*:15, 1968.

Sano, T., Ohshima, H., Tsuchihashi, H., *et al.*: The quantitative analysis of vectorcardiogram of normal hearts and left ventricular hypertrophy. Jap. Heart J., *1*:226, 1960.

Sano, T., Hellerstein, H. K., and Vayda, E.: P vector loop in health and disease as studied by the technique of electrical dissection of the vectorcardiogram (differential vectorcardiography). Am. Heart J., *53*:854, 1957.

Scheuer, J., Kahn, M., Bleifer, S., *et al.*: The atrial vectorcardiogram in health and disease. Am. Heart J., *60*:33, 1960.

Taymor, R. C., Hoffman, I., and Henry, E.: The Frank vectorcardiogram in mitral stenosis. A study of 29 cases. Circulation, *30*:865, 1964.

Toole, J. G., von der Groeben, J., and Spivack, A. P.: The calculated temperospatial heart vector in proved isolated left ventricular overwork. Am. Heart J., *63*:537, 1962.

Toyama, S., Suzuki, K., Ishiyama, T., *et al.*: Vectorcardiographic criteria of left and right ventricular hypertrophy with the Frank system. Jap. Circ. J., *30*:189, 1966.

Upshaw, C. B., Jr.: Simplified clinically applicable vectorcardiographic diagnosis of left ventricular hypertrophy (Frank lead system), Am. Heart J., *74*:749, 1967.

Varriale, P., Alfenito, J. C., and Kennedy, R. J.: The vectorcardiogram of left ventricular hypertrophy. Analysis and criteria (Frank lead system). Circulation, *33*:569, 1966.

Wallace, A. G., McCall, B. W., and Estes, E. H., Jr.: The vectorcardiogram in left ventricular hypertrophy. A study using the Frank lead system. Am. Heart J., *63*:466, 1962.

Walsh, T. J., Roman, G. T., Jr., and Massie, E.: The vectorcardiographic QRSsE-loop findings in chronic cor pulmunale. Am. Heart J., *60*:592, 1960.

Ventricular conduction defects

Baydar, I. D., Walsh, T. J., and Massie, E.: A vectorcardiographic study of right bundle branch block with the Frank lead system. Clinical correlation in ventricular hypertrophy and chronic pulmonary disease. Am. J. Cardiol., *15*:185, 1965.

Becker, R. A., Scher, A. M., and Erickson, R. V.: Ventricular excitation in experimental left bundle branch block. Am. Heart J., *55*:547, 1958.

Bleifer, S., Kahn, M., Grishman, A., *et al.*: Wolff-Parkinson-White Syndrome. A vectorcardiographic, electrocardiographic and clinical study. Am. J. Cardiol., *4*:321, 1959.

Burch, G. E., and DePasquale, N. P.: Electrocardiographic and vectorcardiographic detection of heart disease in the presence of the pre-excitation syndrome (Wolff-Parkinson-White syndrome). Ann. Intern. Med., *54*:387, 1961.

Cabrera, E., Garcia-Font, R., Gaxiola, A., and Pileggi, F.: The vectorcardiogram of ventricular activation in chronic coronary heart disease. Am. Heart J., *55*:557, 1958.

Castellanos, A., Jr., Lemberg, L., Ioannides, G., *et al.*: The vectorcardiogram in right bundle branch block coexisting with left ventricular focal block. Am. J. Cardiol., *18*:705, 1966.

Chou, T-C., and Helm, R. A.: Clinical Vectorcardiography. New York, Grune & Stratton, 1967.

Chung, K-Y., Walsh, T. J., and Massie, E.: Wolff-Parkinson-White syndrome. Am. Heart J., *69*:116, 1965.

Dodge, H. T., and Grant, R. P.: Mechanisms of QRS complex prolongation in man. Am. J. Med., *21*:534, 1956.

Doucet, P., Walsh, T. J., and Massie, E.: A vectorcardiographic study of right bundle branch block with the Frank lead system. Am. J. Cardiol., *16*:342, 1965.

Erickson, R. V., Scher, A. M., and Becker, R. A.: Ventricular excitation in experimental bundle branch block. Circ. Res., *5*:5, 1957.

Frimpter, G. W., Scherr, L., and Ogden, D.: The spatial vectorcardiogram in complete left bundle branch block with special reference to the initial component. Am. Heart J., *55*:220, 1958.

Gambou, R., Penaloza, D., Francisco, S., *et al.*: The role of the right and left ventricles in the ventricular pre-excitation (WPW) syndrome. Am. J. Cardiol., *10*:650, 1962.

Gardberg, M. and Rosen, I. L.: The electrocardiogram and vectorcardiogram in various degrees of left bundle branch block. Am. J. Cardiol., *1*:592, 1958.

Kennamer, R., and Prinzmetal, M.: Depolarization of the ventricle with bundle branch block. Studies on the mechanism of ventricular activity. X. Am. Heart J., *47*:769, 1954.

Luna, R., and Jackson, A.: The vectorcardiogram in left bundle branch block. Am. J. Cardiol., *7*:638, 1961.

Neuman, J., Blackaller, J., Tobin, J. R., *et al.*: The spatial vectorcardiogram in left bundle branch block. Am. J. Cardiol., *16*:352, 1965.

Penaloza, D., Gamboa, R., and Sime, F.: Experimental right bundle branch block in the normal human heart. Electrocardiographic, vectorcardiographic and hemodynamic observation. Am. J. Cardiol., *8*:767, 1961.

Rodriguez, M. I., and Sodi-Pallares, D.: The mechanism of complete and incomplete bundle branch block. Am. Heart J., *44*:715, 1952.

Sanchez, C., Walsh, T. J., and Massie, E.: The vectorcardiogram in incomplete left bundle branch block. Am. J. Cardiol., *7*:629, 1961.

Scherlis, L., and Lee, Y-C.: Right bundle branch block following open heart surgery. Electrocardiographic and vectorcardiographic study. Am. J. Cardiol., 8:780, 1961.

Scherlis, L., and Lee, Y-C: Transient right bundle branch block. An electrocardiographic and vectorcardiographic study. Am. J. Cardiol., 11:173, 1963.

Scott, R.: Left bundle branch block. A clinical assessment. Am. Heart J., 70:535, 1965.

Wallace, A. G., Estes, E. H., and McCall, B. W.: The vectorcardiographic findings in left bundle branch block. A study using the Frank lead system. Am. Heart J., 63:508, 1962.

Myocardial infarction, injury and ischemia

Benchimal, A., and Barreto, E. C.: Serial vectorcardiograms with the Frank system in patients with acute inferior wall myocardial infarction. J. Electrocardiol., 2:159, 1969.

Chou, T-C., and Helm, R. A.: Clinical Vectorcardiography. New York, Grune & Stratton, 1967.

DePasquale, N., and Burch, G. E.: The spatial vectorcardiogram in left bundle branch block and myocardial infarction, with autopsy studies. Am. J. Med., 29:633, 1960.

Doucet, P., Walsh, T. J., and Massie, E.: A vectorcardiographic study of right bundle branch block with the Frank lead system. Clinical correlation in myocardial infarction. Am. J. Cardiol., 16:342, 1965.

Doucet, P., Walsh, T. J., and Massie, E.: A vectorcardiographic and electrocardiographic study of left bundle branch block with myocardial infarction. Am. J. Cardiol., 17:171, 1966.

First, S. R., Bayley, R. H., and Bedford, D. R.: Peri-infarction block; electrocardiographic abnormality occasionally resembling bundle branch block and local ventricular block of other types. Circulation, 2:31, 1950.

Grant, R. P.: Peri-infarction block. Prog. Cardiov. Dis., 2:237, 1959.

Gunnar, R. M., Pietras, R. J., Blackaller, J., et al.: Correlation of vectorcardiographic criteria for myocardial infarction with autopsy findings. Circulation, 35:158, 1967.

Hoffman, I., Taymor, R. C., and Gootnick, A.: Vectorcardiographic residua of inferior infarction. Seventy-eight cases studied with the Frank system. Circulation, 29:562, 1964.

Hoffman, I., Taymor, R. C., Morris, M. H., et al.: Quantitative criteria for the diagnosis of dorsal infarction using the Frank vectorcardiogram. Am. Heart J., 70:295, 1965.

Howitt, G., and Lawrie, T. D. V.: The vectorcardiogram in myocardial infarction. Brit. Heart J., 22:61, 1960.

Hugenholtz, P. G., Ryan, T. J., Woerner, T., et al.: Recognition of anterior wall infarction in patients with left ventricular hypertrophy. A study of the Frank vectorcardiogram. Circulation, 27:386, 1963.

Hugenholtz, P. G., Whipple, G. H., and Levine, H. D.: A clinical appraisal of the vectorcardiogram in myocardial infarction. I. The cube system. Circulation, 24:808, 1961.

Hugenholtz, P. G., Forkner, C. E., Jr., and Levine, H. D.: A clinical appraisal of the vectorcardiogram in myocardial infarction. II. The Frank system. Circulation, 24:825, 1961.

Jacobson, E. D., Rush, S., Zinberg, S., et al.: The effect of infarction on magnitude and orientation of electrical events in the heart. Am. Heart J., 58:863, 1959.

Karni, H.: The TsE loop in myocardial lesions. Am. Heart J., 52:867, 1956.

Libanoff, A. J., Boiteau, G. M., and Allenstein, B. J.: Diaphragmatic myocardial infarction with peri-infarction block. Studies of the electrocardiogram and vectorcardiogram. Am. J. Cardiol., 12:772, 1963.

Mathur, V. S., and Levine, H. D.: Vectorcardiographic differentiation between right ventricular hypertrophy and posterobasal myocardial infarction. Am. J. Cardiol., 17:131, 1966.

Mayer, J. W., Castellanos, A., Jr., and Lemberg, L.: The spatial vectorcardiogram in peri-infarction block. Am. J. Cardiol., 11:613, 1963.

Murata, K., Matsushita, S., Kurihara, H., et al.: Some pitfalls of vectorcardiographic diagnosis of myocardial infarction with particular respect to emphysema. Circulation, 35:172, 1967.

Rothfeld, E. L., Bernstein, A., Wachtel, F., et al.: The vectorcardiogram in direct posterior wall myocardial infarction. Am. J. Cardiol., 10:496, 1961.

Selvester, R. H., Rubin, H. B., Hamlin, J. A., et al.: New quantitative vectorcardiographic criteria for the detection of unsuspected myocardial infarction in diabetics. Am. Heart J., 75:335, 1968.

Toutouzas, P., Hubner, P., Sainani, G., et al.: Value of vectorcardiogram in diagnosis of posterior and inferior myocardial infarctions. Brit. Heart J., 31:629, 1969.

Walsh, T. J., Tiongson, P. M., Stoddard, E. A.: The vectorcardiographic QRSsE-loop findings in infero posterior myocardial infarction. Am. Heart J., 63:516, 1962.

Wolff, L., Wolff, R., Samartzis, M. D., et al.: Vectorcardiographic diagnosis. A correlation with autopsy findings in 167 cases. Circulation, 23:861, 1961.

Miscellaneous VCG patterns

Bahl, O. P., Walsh, T. J., and Massie, E.: Left axis deviation. An electrocardiographic study with post-mortem correlation. Brit. Heart J., 31:451, 1969.

Banta, H. D., Greenfield, J. C., and Estes, E. H., Jr.: Left axis deviation. Am. J. Cardiol., 14:330, 1964.

Blackburn, H., and a Committee: The exercise electrocardiogram. Differences in interpretation. Am. J. Cardiol., 21:871, 1968.

Blackburn, H. (ed.): Measurement in Exercise Electrocardiography. Springfield, Ill., Charles C Thomas, 1969.

Blomqvist, G.: The Frank lead exercise electrocardiogram. Acta Med. Scand., 440 (suppl.), 1965.

Borun, E. R., Chapman, J. M., and Massey, F. J.: Electrocardiographic data recorded with Frank leads. Am. J. Cardiol., 18:656, 1966.

Bruce, R. A., Mazzarella, J. A., Jordan, J. W., et al.: Quantitation of QRS and ST segment responses to exercise. Am. Heart J., 71:455, 1966.

Chou, T-C., Helm, R. A., and Cach, R.: The significance of a wide TsE loop. Circulation, 30:400, 1964.

Isaacs, A., et al.: Ischemic T loop. J. Electrocardiol., 1:68, 1968.

Karni, H.: The TsE loop in myocardial lesions. Am. Heart J., 52:867, 1956.

Master, A. M., and Rosenfeld, I.: Two-step test: current status after twenty-five years. Mod. Conc. Cardiov. Dis., 36:4, 1967.

Pryor, R., and Blount, S. G., Jr.: The clinical significance of true left axis deviation. Left intraventricular blocks. Am. Heart J., 72:391, 1966.

Differentiation between normal and abnormal vectorcardiograms

Chernoff, H., and Moses, L. E.: Elementary Decision Theory. New York, John Wiley & Sons, 1959.

Feinstein, A. R.: Clinical Judgment. Baltimore, Williams & Wilkins, 1967.

Freund, J. E.: Modern Elementary Statistics. Englewood Cliffs, N. J., Prentice-Hall, Inc., 1967.

Lusted, L. B.: Introduction to Medical Decision Making. Springfield, Ill., Charles C Thomas Publisher, 1968.

Mode, E. B.: Elements of Probability and Statistics. Englewood Cliffs, N. J., Prentice-Hall, Inc., 1966.

Schlaifer, R.: Probability and Statistics for Business Decisions. New York, McGraw-Hill, 1959.

Simonson, E.: Differentiation Between Normal and Abnormal in Electrocardiography. St. Louis, C. V. Mosby, 1961.

Wartak, J.: An information theory approach to medical diagnosis. Cybernetica, 3:162, 1965.

Wartak, J.: ECG criteria for angina pectoris derived from resting Frank lead electrocardiograms. Chest, 58:42, 1970.

Wartak, J., and Milliken, J. A.: A logical approach to diagnosing electrocardiograms. J. Electrocardiol., 2:337, 1969.

Interpretation of the vectorcardiogram

Burch, G. E., Abildskov, J. A., and Cronvich, J. A.: Vectorcardiography. Circulation, 8:605, 1953.

Burch, G. E., Golden, L. H., and Cronvich, J. A.: An analysis of changes in spatial vectorcardiogram with aging. Am. Heart J., 55:582, 1958.

Emslie-Smith, D., and Lowe, K. G.: The spatial vectorcardiogram in diagnosis. Postgrad. Med. J., 8:39, 1968.

Geselowitz, D. B.: Dipole theory in electrocardiography. Am. J. Cardiol., 14, 301, 1964.

Heckert, E. W., Cook, W. R., and Krause, S.: The clinical value of vectorcardiography. Am. J. Cardiol., 7:657, 1961.

Hugenholtz, P. G., Forkner, C. E., and Levine, H. D.: A clinical appraisal of the vectorcardiogram in myocardial infarction. II. The Frank system. Circulation, 24:825, 1961.

Johnston, F. D.: The clinical value of vectorcardiography. Circulation, 23:297, 1961.

Okada, R. H.: A critical review of vector electrocardiography. IEEE Trans. Biomed. Electronics, 10:95, 1963.

Prinzmetal, M., et al.: Clinical implications of errors in electrocardiographic diagnosis: Heart disease of electrocardiographic origin. JAMA, 161:138, 1956.

Skowron, A.: Examination of the validity of the concept of vectorcardiography. Brit. Heart J., 30:735, 1968.

Schmitt, O. H., and Simonson, E.: The present status of vectorcardiography. Arch. Intern. Med., 96:574, 1955.

Simonson, E., et al.: Diagnostic accuracy of the vectorcardiogram and electrocardiogram. A cooperative study. Am. J. Cardiol., 17:829, 1966.

Sotobata, I., Richman, H., and Simonson, E.: Sex differences in the vectorcardiogram. Circulation, 37:438, 1968.

Woods, J. D., Laurie, W., and Smith, W. G.: The reliability of the electrocardiogram in myocardial infarction. Lancet, 2:265, 1963.

Computer assisted interpretation of VCGs

Caceres, C. A.: A basis for observer variation in electrocardiographic interpretation. Prog. in Cardiov. Dis., 5:521, 1963.

Caceres, C. A., et al.: Computer aids in electrocardiography. Ann. N. Y. Acad. Sci., 118:85, 1964.

Cooper, J. K., et al.: Role of a digital computer in a diagnostic center. JAMA, 193:911, 1965.

Dobrow, R. J., et al.: Accuracy of electrocardiographic measurements by a computer system. Am. J. Med. Electronics, 4:121, 1965.

King, P. J. H.: Decision tables. Comp. Journal, 10:135, 1967.

McDaniel, H.: An Introduction to Decision Logic Tables. New York, John Wiley & Sons, 1968.

Milliken, J. A., and Wartak, J., (eds.): Computers and Electrocardiography. Proceedings of the Workshop held at Queen's University, October 3–4, 1968, Queen's University, Kingston, Canada.

Milliken, J. A., Wartak, J., Orme, W., et al.: Use of computers in the interpretation of electrocardiograms. Canad. Med. Ass. J., 101:377, 1969.

Mori, H., et al.: Spatial analytico-geometrical analysis of the vectorcardiogram by electronic computer. Jap. Circ. J., 30:1017, 1966.

Okajima, M., et al.: Computer pattern recognition techniques: some results with real electrocardiographic data. IEEE Trans. Biomed. Electronics, 10:106, 1963.

Press, L. I.: Conversion of decision tables to computer programs. Comm. ACM, 8:385, 1965.

Smith, R. E., and Hyde, C. M.: A computer system for electrocardiographic analysis. Proc. of the Third Annual Rocky Mountain Bio-Engineering Symposium, Univ. of Colorado, Boulder, Colorado, May 1966.

Stallmann, F. W.: A computer program for automatic analysis of electrocardiograms. Am. Heart J., 67:136, 1964.

Stark, L.: Pattern recognition for electrocardiographic diagnosis. M.I.T. Research Lab. of Electronics. Cambridge, Mass., Quart. Prog. Rept. No. 61, May 1960.

Stark, L., Dickson, J. F., Whipple, G. H., and Horibe, H.: Remote real-time diagnosis of clinical electrocardiograms by a digital computer. Ann. N. Y. Acad. Sci., 128:851, 1966.

Vienott, C. G.: Programming decision tables in FORTRAN, COBOL or ALGOL. Comm. ACM, 9:31, 1966.

Vienott, C. G.: Decision tables education guide. Form R25–1684, IBM Corp., 1962.

Wartak, J.: Computer-aided recognition of electrocardiograms. Acta Cardiol., 22:350, 1967.

Wartak, J.: A practical approach to automated diagnosis. IEEE Trans. Biomed. Electronics Eng., 17:37, 1970.

Wartak, J.: Computers in Electrocardiography. Springfield, Ill., Charles C Thomas, 1970.

Wartak, J., and Milliken, J. A.: Logical approach to diagnosing electrocardiograms. J. Electrocardiol., 2:337, 1969.

Wartak, J., and Milliken, J. A.: Computer analysis of the ECG data using decision tables techniques. Proceedings of the DECUS Symposium, Las Vegas, Nov. 17–18, 1969, p. 425.

Index

Numerals in italics indicate a diagram, "t" following a page number indicates a table, on the subject mentioned.

Age, chronological, as influence on vectorcardiogram, 160
Amplifiers, of electrocardiograph, 40, *40*
Angina pectoris, diagnosis of, exercise tests for, 132-134, *132, 133*
    vectorcardiogram in, 134, *134*
    origin of, 132
Angle, azimuth, 50
    QRS-T, 60, *60*
        normal range of, 130, *130*
Angular scale, 51, *51*
Arithmetic mean, in statistical analysis of vectorcardiogram, 141-142, *141, 142*
Atom(s), 2, *2*
Atrium(a), left, enlargement of, electrocardiogram in, 92, *92*
        vectorcardiogram in, 92, *92*
    normal, vectorcardiogram in, 90, *90*
    right, enlargement of, electrocardiogram in, 91, *91*
        vectorcardiogram in, 90, 91, *91*
Average(s), arithmetic, 141, *141*
    median, 142, *142*
    mode, 142, *142*
Axis, left, of heart, deviation of, 128-129, *128, 129*

Bayes theorem, in probability calculations, 172
"Bite-out," in vectorcardiogram loop, 116, *116*
Bundle branch block, left, conditions causing, 104
    electrocardiogram in, 106, *106*
    origin of, 104, *104*
    vectorcardiogram in, 104-105, *104, 105*
    right, conditions causing, 107
    electrocardiogram in, 109, *109*
    origin of, 107, *107*
    vectorcardiogram in, 107-109, *107, 108*
    vectorcardiogram pattern demonstrating, 85, *85*
Burger triangle, 37, *37*
    hexaxial system based on, 62, *62*

Cardiac dipole. *See* Dipole, cardiac
Cartesian coordinate system, in plane, 18, *18*
    in 3-dimensional space, 19, *19*
Cell(s), cardiac, activation of, 6-7, *7, 8*
    damaged, injury potential in, 6, *6*
    depolarized, 6, *7*
    ionic balance of, restoration of, 6, *7*
    polarized, 6, *6*
    repolarized, 6, *7*
    resting state of, 6
Central tendency, measures of, 141-142
Charge(s), electrical, 2
    negative, electrical field surrounding, 3, *3*

Charge(s)—(*Cont.*)
    positive, electrical field surrounding, 3, *3*
Chest, configuration of, as influence on vectorcardiogram, 161
Classification, of vectorcardiogram, statistical technique of, 148, *148*
Components X, Y, and Z, analysis of, 52-54
Computer, in interpretation of vectorcardiograms, 162-172
    vectorcardiographic data for, acquisition cart collecting, 164, *164*
    coding of, 164, *164*
    processing of, 162-163, *163*
    recorded on magnetic tape, 165, *165*
    vectorcardiogram diagnosis by, decision tables in, 170-171
    probability calculus in, 172, *172*
    vectorcardiographic waveform, recognized by, 166-169, *166, 167, 168, 169*
Conduction defects, ventricular, 104-113
Conduction system, of heart, 8, *8*
Conductor, volume, 11
    electrical potential in, law governing, 12, *13*
    human body as, 12, 13
Constitution, body, variables of, influence on vectorcardiogram, 161
Coordinate system, orthogonal, new, 25
    polar, in 3-dimensional space, 22, *22*
Coordinates, polar, definition of, 50
    of heart vector, on horizontal plane, 50, *50*
        in 3-dimensional space, 50, *50*
    rectangular, planes formed by, 49, *49*
        for recording of spatial heart vector, 49, *49*
Cube lead system, 35, *35*
Current, dipole, 6-7
    electric, 4-5
    alternating, 5, *5*
    direct, 5
    flow of, in electrolyte solution, 5, *5*
        in flashlight battery, *5*
        in metal wire, 5, *5*
Current field, electrical, pattern of, generated by dipole, 12, *12*
    surrounding cardiac dipole, 12
    surrounding dipole, recording of difference between points in, 12, *12*

Decision tables, in diagnosis of vectorcardiogram by computer, 170-171, *171*
    mechanics of using, 171, *171*
    structure of, 170, *170*
Decision tree structure, in logical data evaluation, 138, *138*
Deflections, electrocardiographic, amplitude and polarity of, 52, *52*
    terminology of, 52-54, *53*

Depolarization, cardiac, of muscle fiber, 6, *7*
    process of, 8
    spread of, 8, *9*
    dipole in stages of, 8, *10*
    ventricular, instantaneous vectors representing, 26, *26*
    and resultant cardiac dipoles, 10, *10*
    vectors of, grouped, 78, *78*
Deviation, mean, calculation of, 143, *143*
    standard, calculation of, 143, *143*
Digitalis, producing ST-T vector changes, 130, *130*
Dipole, cardiac, composition of, 11, *11*
    concept of, 10-13
    in vectorcardiography, importance of, 157-159, *158*
    electrical field surrounding, 12
    geometry of, 20-28
    origin of, 10
    physics of, 11-12
    represented by vector, 11, *11*
    and ventricular depolarization, 10, *10*
    current, 6-7
    vector representation of, 11, *11*
    voltage induced by, law governing, 12, *13*
    in volume conductor, 11-12, *12*
    pattern of current field generated by, 12, *12*
Disease, cardiac. *See* Heart disease
Dispersion, measures of, 142-143
    96 percentile range, 142, *142*
    range of data, 140, *142*
Distribution curve, normal, as representation of relative frequency, 144, *144*
    in statistical analysis of vectorcardiogram, 145, *145*

Eigenvectors, 25
Einthoven, lead system of, 36-37, *37*, 39, *39*, 61, *61*
Electric current. *See* Current, electric
Electrical activity, of heart. *See* Heart, electrical activity of
Electricity, charges of, 2
    concepts of, fundamental, 2-5
    current of, 4-5
    field of, 3
    potentials of, 4
Electrocardiogram, 52-54, *53, 54*
    intervals of, 54, *54*
    orthogonal, 23
    segments of, 54, *54*
    12 lead, 39, 56
    analysis of, 61-63
    frontal plane leads of, 61-62, *61, 62*
    horizontal plane leads of, 62, *63*
    normal, 78-81
    data, statistical characteristics of, 80t, 81, 81t, *81*

Electrocardiogram—(*Cont.*)
    patterns, genesis of, 78-79, *78, 79*
    and vectorcardiogram, combined interpretation of, 159, *159*
    waves of, 53, *53*
Electrocardiograph, 46-48
    amplifiers of, 40, *40*
    deflections of, analysis of, 52, *52*
        terminology of, 52-54, *53*
    direct-writing, components of, 46, *46*
    frequency distortion of wave of, 40, *40*
    optical, components of, 47, *47*
    signal conditioning in, 40, *40*
    standard grid of, 48, *48*
    standardization of, 48, *48*
    strip chart record of, 48
    types of, compared, 47
Electrocardiographic patterns, normal, data in, statistical characteristics of, 80t, 81, 81t, *81*
    genesis of, 78-79, *78, 79*
Electrocardiography, mean vectors, calculation in, 26-27
    of ventricular depolarization analyzed, 27
    ventricular gradient vector in, 27-28
Electrons, 2, *2*
Equipotential lines, 4, *4*
Errors, diagnostic, false-negative, 149, *149*
    false-positive, 149, *149*
Exercise tests, vectorcardiogram in, 132-134, *134*

Field, electric, 3
    difference of electrical potential in, 4, *4*
    surrounding electrical charges, 3, *3*
Force, of attraction (or repulsion), 2, *2*
    field of, 3
        difference of electric potential in, 4, *4*
    gravitational, surrounding earth, 3, *3*
Frank, lead system of, 33-34, *33, 34,* 64-65
    electrode placement in, 33, *33*
    image vectors for, 33, *34*
    polarity of leads in, 33-34, *34*
    resistor network for, 33, *33*
Frequency curve, to depict distribution of data, 144, *144*
Frequency distribution tables, in statistical grouping of data, 140, *140*
Frequency polygon, in statistical analysis of data, 141, *141*

Goldberger, unipolar limb leads, augmented by, 38-39, *39*
Gravity, 3
    field of, surrounding earth, *3*

Heart, abnormalities of, diagnosis of, 82
    activation in, electrical state of, 6-7
        spread of, 8
    cells of. *See* Cell(s), cardiac
    conduction defect of, ventricular, vectorcardiogram pattern demonstrating, 85, *85*
    conduction system of, 8, *8*
    disease of. *See* Heart disease
    electrical activity of, 2-13

Heart—(*Cont.*)
    abnormal patterns of, 82-87
    dipole in. *See* Dipole, cardiac
    instruments recording, 40-48
    lead systems for recording, 29-39
    methods of analyzing, 49-63
    normal patterns of, 64-81
    electrical forces of, vector representation of, 15-28
    electricity of, ionic basis of, 6-9
    left axis deviation of, clinical significance of, 128, *128*
        electrocardiogram in, 129, *129*
        vectorcardiogram in, 129, *129*
    resting, electrical state of, 6
    hypertrophy of, vectorcardiogram pattern demonstrating, 84, *84,* 90-103
    myocardial infarction of, vectorcardiogram pattern demonstrating, 86-87, *86, 87*
    vectors. *See* Vector(s), heart
Heart disease, diagnosis of, errors in, 149
    diagnostic criteria in, reliability of, 151
        selection of, 150
    vectorcardiogram in, 90-134
Hexaxial system, in analysis of electrocardiogram, *61,* 62, *62*
Histogram, in statistical grouping of data, 140-141, *140,* 144, *144*
Hypertrophy, biventricular, diagnostic features of, 103
    diseases causing, 102
    vectorcardiogram in, 102-103, *102, 103*
    ventricular. *See* Ventricle(s), hypertrophy of

Image space, and lead vectors, 30, *30*
Infarction, myocardial. *See* Myocardial infarction
Intensity, electrical, 3, *3*
Intervals, of electrocardiogram, 54, *54*
Ion(s), 2, *2*
Ischemia, local, producing ST-T vector changes, 131, *131*

Kirchhoff's law, 36, *36*

Latitude, geographic lines of, *50*
Lead(s), axis(es), definition of, 29, *29*
        discrepancies in, 29, *29*
    definition of, 29
    electrocardiographic, physical and mathematical properties of, 29-32
    frontal plane, 61-62, *61, 62*
    horizontal plane, 62, *63*
    limb, bipolar, 36, *36*
        standard, 36-37
    orthogonal, axes of, system of, 49, *49*
        corrected, 31-32, *32*
    precordial, axes of, in horizontal plane, 39, *39*
    strength of, variation in, 29, *29*
    unipolar, 38-39
        augmented by Goldberger, 38-39, *39*
        of Wilson, 38, *38*
    vectorial concept of, 30
Lead system(s), with axes mutually perpendicular and of equal scale, 29, *29*
    cube, 35, *35*
    Frank, 33-34, *33, 34,* 64-65
    orthogonal, 22, 33-35

Lead system(s)—(*Cont.*)
    for recording electrical activity of heart, 29-39
    tetrahedron, 34-35, *35*
    twelve, 36-39, 61-63
    uncorrected vector, 34-35
Lead vectors. *See* Vector(s), lead
Lines, equipotential, 4, *4*
    of field intensity, 3, *3*
    of force, 3, *3,* 4, *4*
    potential, 4
Logic, role of, in diagnosis of vectorcardiograms, 137-139, *137*
Longitude, geographic lines of, *50*
Loop(s), spatial, calculation of three axes of, 25, *25*
    of heart vector, 24-25
        formation of, 21, *21*
        plane of predilection, 24, *24*
    vector, analysis of, 55-60
        construction of, 55-56, *55, 56*
        P, 56, *57,* 72, *72*
        QRS, 56-59, *57, 58, 59,* 73-75, *73, 74, 75*
            configuration of, 57-59, *58*
            inscription of, direction and speed of, 57, *57*
            magnitude and direction of, 59, *59*
        T, 60, *60*
    three dimensional, by generating cones at different angles, 42, *42*
        by modulation of horizontal vector loop, 42, *42*
        by stereo effect, 42, *42*
    vectorcardiographic, angular velocity of inscription of, 24, *24*
        "bite-out" of, 116, *116*
        dashes of, interpretation of, 41
        definition of, 23
        descriptions of, 156
        in heart disorders. *See Specific disorders*
        linear velocity of inscription of, 23-24, *23*
        oscilloscope displaying, 41, *41*
        rotation of, 44, *44*

Master two-step test, in diagnosis of angina pectoris, 132, *132, 133*
Mean deviation, calculation of, in statistical analysis of vectorcardiogram, 143, *143*
Muscle fiber, of heart, depolarization of, 6, *7*
    ionic balance in, restoration of, 6, *7*
    polarized state of, at rest, 6
    repolarization of, 6, *7*
    transitional zone of, as site of microscopic dipoles, 7, *8*
Myocardial infarction, acute, 6
    anterior, electrocardiogram in, 121, *121*
        site of, 119, *119*
        vectorcardiogram in, 120-121, *120, 121*
    diagnosis of, 115
    extent of, classified, 119, *119*
    inferoposterior (posterodiaphragmatic), electrocardiogram, in 125, *125*

Myocardial infarction—(*Cont.*)
    site of, 119, *119*
    vectorcardiogram in, 124-125, *124,
      125*
  lateral, electrocardiogram in, 123, *123*
    site of, 119, *119*
    vectorcardiogram in, 122-123, *122,
      123*
  pathogenesis of, 114-115
  true posterior, electrocardiogram in,
    126, *126*
    site of, 119, *119*
    vectorcardiogram in, 126, *126*
  vectorcardiogram in, 114-126
  vectorcardiogram changes in, rare, 116,
    116
    typical, 115-116, *115, 116*
  vectorcardiogram charting course of,
    117, *117*
  vectorcardiogram pattern demonstrat-
    ing, 86-87, *86, 87*
  vectorcardiogram to predict location of
    infarct, 118-119, *118*

Orthogonal coordinate system, new, 25
Oscilloscope, cathode-ray tube of, 41
  scalar tracing from, 41, *41*
  teardrop-shaped dashes of, 41, *42*
  vectorcardiogram loop from, 41, *42*

P vector loop, 56, 72, *72*
Parallelogram law, in addition of vectors,
  17, *17*
Peri-infarction block, occurrence of, 127
  vectorcardiogram in, 127, *127*
Polar coordinate system, in 3-dimensional
  space, 22, *22*
Polar vector, in vectorcardiography, 24-
  25, *24*
Polarcardiogram, 23, 44
Polarcardiograph, 44-46
  principle of operation of, 44-45, *44*
  time plots of polar coordinates, 45-46,
    45
  advantages of, 46
Polarization, of myocardial fiber, 6, *6*
Potential, cardiac, of action, 6-7
  transmembrane, 6
  electric, 4
Probability, calculation of, in evaluation
  of vectorcardiogram, 152-153, *153*
Probability density, joint, calculation of,
  172, *172*
Protons, 2, *2*

QRS vector loop, 57-59, *57, 58, 59,* 73-
  75, *73, 74, 75*
QRS-T angle, 60, *60*
  normal range of, 130, *130*

Race, influence of, on vectorcardiogram,
  161
Repolarization, cardiac, of muscle fiber,
  6, *7*
  process of, 7
  spread of, 7, 8
Reports, of vectorcardiogram findings,
  154-156
Resistance, to current flow, 5
  measurement of, 5

Resolver, 43-44
  rotation of vectorcardiographic loops
    by, 44, *44*
  transformation of coordinates by, 43,
    43

Scalar(s), becoming vector, pictorial con-
  cept of, *19*
  in projection of two vectors, 20
  versus vectors, 15
Scalarcardiogram, 23
Scale, angular, 51, *51*
Segments, of electrocardiograms, 54, *54*
Sensitivity, as diagnostic criterion in heart
  disease, 151, *151*
Sex, influence of, vectorcardiogram, 161
Sino-atrial node, as pacemaker, 8
Sodium pump, 7
Specificity, as diagnostic criterion in heart
  disease, 151, *151*
Standard deviation, calculation of, in
  statistical analysis of vectorcardiogram,
  143, *143*
Statistics, role of, in analysis of vector-
  cardiograms, 140-145
Symbols, in heart vector notation, 21-22

T vector loop, 60, *60*
Terminal, central, of Wilson, 38, *38*
Tetrahedron lead system, 34-35, *35*
Treadmill, motor-driven, in diagnosis of
  angina pectoris, 133, *133*
Triangle(s), Burger scalene, 37, *37*
  hexaxial system based on, 62, *62*
  Einthoven equilateral, 36-37, *37,* 39,
    39, 61, *61*
Triangle hypothesis, of Einthoven, 36-37,
  37
Trigonometry, elements of, formulas de-
  fining, 20
  functions of, geometrical representa-
    tion of, *20*

Values, vectorcardiographic, normal, 146-
  147
Variability, measures of, 142-143
Variables, constitutional, influence on
  vectorcardiogram, 160, 161
Vector(s), analysis of elements of, 15-20
  atrial repolarization, 56, *57*
  cardiac, direction of, in plane, 51, *51*
  changes of, in atrial enlargement, 90-
    92, *90*
    causes of, 83
    classification of, by ventricular gradi-
      ent concept, 83
    in hypertrophy of heart, 84, *84,* 90-
      103
    in myocardial infarction, 86-87, *86,
      87*
    nonspecific, in ST-T vectors, 130-
      131
    in ventricular conduction defect of
      heart, 85, *85*
  coordinates of, in plane, 18-19, *18*
    in 3-dimensional space, 19, *19*
  decomposition of, 18-19
  definition of, 15
  depolarization of ventricles represented
    by, 8, *10,* 10-11
  designation of, in text, 15, *15*

Vector(s)—(*Cont.*)
  dipole represented by, 11, *11*
  geometrical representation of, *15*
  heart, concept of, 20-21, *20*
    frontal plane, resolved into scalar
      components, *22*
    instantaneous, 26, *26*
      averaging of, 26
      maximal, 26, *26*
    and lead vector, scalar product of,
      30, *30*
    mean, 26-28, *26*
      calculated, 26-27, *27*
      magnitude of, calculated, 27
      orientation of, calculation of, 27
      of ventricular depolarization, an-
        alyzed, 27, *27*
    mean distance to plane of predilec-
      tion, calculation of, 25, *25*
    notation of, 21-22
    orientation and magnitude of, *52*
    plane projection of, 23-24, *22, 23*
    polar coordinate system defining, 22
    reconstruction of, 29
    resultant, 26, *26*
    scalar components of, 22-23
    spatial, magnitude of, computation
      of, 22
      resolved into scalar components,
        22, *22*
    spatial loops of, 21, 24-25
      and planar projections, *21*
    symbols for notation of, 21-22
  lead, definition of, 30
    dipole location, insensitivity to, 31-
      32, *32*
    and heart vector, scalar product of,
      30, *30*
    and image space, 30, *30*
    magnitude and direction of, 31, *32*
    measurement of, 31-32, *31, 32*
  length of, calculation of, 19
  loops. *See* Loop(s), vector
  P, spatial, normal, 71, *71*
  polar, 24-25, *24*
  projection of, on plane, 20, *20*
    on line, 20, *20*
  QRS, normal, 73-75
  repolarization of ventricles represented
    by, 7
  as result of sum of individual dipole
    vectors, 7, *8*
  scalar quantity becoming, pictorial con-
    cept of, *19*
  scalars, distinction between, 15
  ST, normal, 75, *75*
  ST-T, nonspecific changes of, condi-
    tions causing, 130
    definition of, 130
    digitalis producing, 130, *130*
    ischemia producing, 131, *131*
  subtraction of, method of, 17, *17*
  sum of, calculation of, 16-17, *16, 17*
  T, normal, 76-77
  two, scalar product of, 20, *20*
  ventricular gradient, calculation of, 27-
    28, *28*
Vectorcardiogram, abnormalities in, assessment of, 82
  classification of, 83
  vector interpretation of, 84, *84*

Vectorcardiogram—(*Cont.*)
 analysis of, logical, 137-139
  statistical, 140-145
 bundle branch block displayed by, 85, *85*
 in cardiac disease, 90-134
 classification of, statistical technique of, 148, *148*
 clinical value of, 157-161
 and computer, data acquisition for, 164-165, *164, 165*
  data processing for, 162-163, *163*
  diagnosis by, 170-172
  interpretation assistance by, 162-172
  waveform recognition by, 166-169, *166, 167, 168, 169*
 constitutional variables, correlation with, 160
 definition of, 23
 diagnosis of, decision tree method in, 138, *139*
  role of logic in, 137-139, *137*
 diagnostic evaluation of, 82, 137-172
 and electrocardiogram, combined interpretation of, 159, *159*
 evaluation of, decision problem in, 148-153
  diagnostic criteria in, 150-151
  diagnostic errors in, 149, *149*
  probability calculation in, 152-153, *152*
 interpretation of, 154-161
 normal, 64-77
  and abnormal, differentiation between, 137-153
  data, appraisal of, 64
   statistical characteristics of 64-70, 65t, *65*, 66t, *66*, 67t, *67*, 68t, *68*, 69t, *69*, 70t, *70*
  left ventricle contributing to, 73, *73*
  P vector of, 71-72
   planar projections of, 72, *72*
   X, Y, Z components, 71, *71*
  QRS vector of, 73-75
   frontal plane of, 74, *74*
   horizontal plane of, 73, *73*
   sagittal plane of, 74-75, *75*

Vectorcardiogram—(*Cont.*)
   X, Y, Z components of, 73, *73*
   ST vector of, 75, *75*
   T vector of, 76-77
    planar projections, 76-77, *76, 77*
    X, Y, Z components, 76, *76*
   values of, 146-147
  patterns of. *See* Vectorcardiographic patterns
  record, *154*
   report of, *155*
  report, form of, 154, *156*
   loop description in, 156
   terminology of, 156
  spatial, 21, *21*
  statistical analysis of, 140-145
  value of, clinical, 157-161
  values of, normal limits of, 147, *147*
  physiological variability in, 146, *146*
  waveform identification, for computer analysis, 166-169, *166, 167, 168, 169*
Vectorcardiograph, diagram of, *41*
 displaying three-dimensional loops, 42
 oscilloscope displaying, 41, *41*
 signal conditioning in, 40
Vectorcardiographic patterns, abnormalities in, assessment of, 82
 classification of, 83
 computer recognition of, 166-169, *168, 169*
 miscellaneous, 128-134
Vectorcardiography, angular scale in, 51, *51*
 heart dipole concept in, importance of, 157-158
 limitations of, 157
 polar coordinates of, 50, *50*
 principles of, 1-87
 rectangular coordinates of, 49, *49*
 reference frame for, 49-51
 terminology used in, 50
Ventricle(s), both, hypertrophy of, diagnostic features of, 103
  diseases causing, 102
  vectorcardiogram in, 102-103, *102, 103*

Ventricle(s)—(*Cont.*)
 conduction defects of, 104-113
 left, hypertrophy of, anatomical changes in, 93, *93*
  diseases causing, 93
  electrocardiogram in, 96, *96*
  vectorcardiogram in, 93-95, *93, 94, 95*
 right, hypertrophy of, dextro-anterior type, electrocardiogram in, 99, *99*
  vectorcardiogram in, 98-99, *98, 99*
  dextro-posterior type, electrocardiogram in, 101, *101*
  vectorcardiogram in, 100-101, *100, 101*
  factors causing, 97, *97*
  vectorcardiogram in, 97-101, *97, 98, 99, 100, 101*
Volt(s), definition of, 4
Voltage, definition of, 4
 induced by dipole, law governing, 12, *13*
 and resistance, 5

Waveform, vectorcardiographic, identification of, for computer analysis, 166-169, *166, 167, 168, 169*
Waves, of electrocardiogram, 53, *53*
Weight, body, as influence on vectorcardiogram, 161
Wilson, central terminal of, 38, *38*
 unipolar precordial leads of, 38, *38*
Wolff-Parkinson-White syndrome, conditions causing, 110
 mechanism underlying, possible, 110, *110*
 type A, electrocardiogram in, 111, *111*
  vectorcardiogram in, 110-111, *110, 111*
 type B, electrocardiogram in, 113, *113*
 type B, vectorcardiogram in, 112-113, *112, 113*

X, Y, and Z Components, analysis of, 52-54